Contents

Caring for someone who has dementia

Jane Brotchie

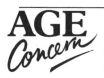

BOOKS

C529327

© 1995 Jane Brotchie
Published by Age Concern England
1268 London Road
London SW16 4ER

First published 1995 in Age Concern Books' *Caring in a Crisis* series
This edition published 1998
Reprinted 1999

Editor Caroline Hartnell
Production Vinnette Marshall
Designed and typeset by GreenGate Publishing Services, Tonbridge, Kent
Printed in Great Britain by Bell & Bain Ltd, Glasgow

A catalogue record for this book is available from the British Library.

ISBN 0-86242-259-0

Bulk orders

Age Concern England is pleased to offer customised editions of all its titles to UK
companies, institutions or other organisations wishing to make a bulk purchase.
For further information, please contact the Publishing Department at the address
above. Tel: 0181-765 7200. Fax: 0181-765 7211. E-mail: addisom@ace.org.uk.

About the author

Jane Brotchie is a freelance author, social researcher and editor. She has worked with young people with learning difficulties and their carers and has also helped to set up carer support projects across East Sussex.

As a writer, Jane has contributed to the national and professional press; she has published a number of research studies and training manuals. Previous books on caring include *Help at Hand: A survival guide for carers* (Bedford Square Press, 1990) and *Equal Shares in Caring* (co-written with Dione Hills, Ruskin College/Socialist Health Association, 1991).

Acknowledgements

Many thanks to: Jean Wooller; Brighton Area Branch of the Alzheimer's Disease Society, particularly Neil McArthur and Tracy Whittle; Gail Elkington at the Carers National Association and *The Carer* magazine; Dr David Jolley, Honorary Reader, Old Age Psychiatry, at Wittington Hospital, Manchester, and Clive Evers of the Alzheimer's Disease Society, for reading and commenting on the first draft; Evelyn McEwen, Jane Whelan, Lorna Easterbrook, Audrey King and Sally West at Age Concern England for their helpful comments; Vinnette Marshall for preparing the typescript; Caroline Hartnell for her editing; all the carers who generously shared their thoughts and experiences with me.

Introduction

Dementia is one of the most common conditions in this country, and one of the least understood. It is also one of the most distressing illnesses for those who develop the condition and for their partners, families and friends.

This book is written for you, the carer. You may be living with the person who has dementia, or you may be living some distance away. You may be the only person providing care, or you may be sharing the care with other members of the family and with professionals.

This book is intended both for those who are facing a crisis now and need information and reassurance and for those who want to plan ahead to prevent a situation developing into a crisis. With a long, slow illness like dementia, a 'crisis' may take different forms: it may build up over time or it may be a moment of sudden shock when, for example, you first realise that your relative may be seriously ill. You are then faced with the difficult question of what you tell your relative if you know or suspect he or she has dementia. A crisis may also arise at a later stage in the illness, perhaps when your relative has a fall and has to go into hospital, and you realise that you cannot go on any longer as you were.

The point when a crisis occurs may depend on whether you are living with the person who has dementia or they live alone. Difficult decisions have to be made when the person has been living alone and it becomes clear that he or she is no longer able to live independently. If you live with the ill person, you may cope for a long time (although quietly compensating for their lost abilities) until the illness takes a new turn and they develop further symptoms such as incontinence or aggression.

Some people with dementia deny that there is anything wrong, which can make caring for them an even more lonely task. Some carers even start to doubt their own sanity.

Whatever your particular circumstances, caring for someone with dementia can be hard, both physically and emotionally. When you are tired, it can be difficult to think what you can do to make your situation easier. This book aims to do some of that work for you: it tells you more about the illness, what to expect in the future, and how to get help now – both for you and for the person you care for. It is based on the experiences of carers themselves who want to help other carers to avoid a crisis in the future that will be painful both for the carer and for the person who is being cared for. The book has also benefited from the long-established expertise of Age Concern and other organisations and professionals who work with people who have dementia.

If you have been caring for some time, you may be feeling isolated and alone. Throughout this book, you will be encouraged to talk to others about your situation and to seek help. Each chapter looks at different points where a crisis can occur and gives you information and ideas about whom to turn to – in the hope that 'to be forewarned is to be forearmed' and that you may be able to prevent a crisis from happening. If there is one message that is repeated again and again by those who have cared for a person with dementia, it is: 'Ask for help early, from as many people as you can, and make sure you have some time away from caring.'

Chapter 1 gives you the information you need when you first realise your relative may have dementia. It explains what we know – and what we don't know – about the illness and how it may develop. It also explains how a diagnosis may be made and how to get medical help. Finally, it looks at the difficult issue of what you tell the person with dementia about their illness.

Chapter 2 addresses some of the important decisions that you, the carer, need to make early on in the illness. You may still be shocked and wondering how you will cope: if you don't know where to start or whom to turn to, this chapter is a guide. Action now may help to avert a crisis later on.

Chapter 3 is for carers who realise that professional help is needed. It describes all the different people and organisations who can provide help and support to you and the person you care for. It also looks at respite care – to give the carer a break from caring – both in the ill person's own home and away from home.

Chapter 4 looks at some of the particular problems of caring for someone in the later stages of dementia. A situation that has been just manageable can suddenly become unbearable. This chapter discusses some of the difficulties that carers often perceive as 'breaking points' in caring. It then goes on to outline the options for alternative care when you have done all you can at home.

Chapter 5 tells you how to plan for the time when your relative is no longer able to manage their own money and affairs. It also outlines the benefits and allowances you and your relative may be able to claim. The financial strain of caring for someone with dementia can be a cause of great worry, but many benefits still go unclaimed.

Chapter 6 describes the impact that caring can have on the carer and other members of the family. The strain of caring can lead to breakdown of relationships and loneliness. Understanding – and accepting – how you and others are feeling can help to strengthen relationships and ensure that you have the support you need.

The person needing care may be a spouse or partner, a parent, sibling or another relative, or a close friend. For simplicity we refer to 'your relative' throughout the book, and 'she' and 'he' in alternate chapters.

> 'The Alzheimer's patient asks nothing more than a hand to hold, a heart to care, and a mind to think for them when they cannot; someone to protect them as they travel through the dangerous twists and turns of the labyrinth.'
>
> Diana Friel McGowin, author of *Living in the Labyrinth* and diagnosed as having Alzheimer's disease

1 Understanding dementia

Tell-tale slips in the behaviour of someone close to you may have alerted you to the possibility that something is wrong. The thought that this might be the onset of dementia is a frightening prospect. A confused state is not necessarily a sign that dementia is beginning, however: it is still possible that the cause of the difficulties is something that can be treated. For this reason, you need to seek help at an early stage.

Some people are relieved to hear a diagnosis of dementia: it may at least provide an explanation for behaviour that they have long found worrying. But if you have not been expecting it, you may be thrown into crisis. You will probably come up with lots of questions that you want answers to. What does it mean? How will I cope? How long will it last? Who will help me? This chapter aims to answer some of these initial questions. It tells you about the symptoms of dementia and the illnesses that cause it and explains how a diagnosis of dementia may be made. Finally, it discusses the difficult question of how much you tell your relative about what is happening to her.

Elsie

'The worst part is in the beginning when you realise there's something wrong.'

1

'He was still working when it started. He used to do the till up and forget where he put the money. He'd go back and find the money gone and say that someone had stolen it. The worst part is in the beginning when you realise there's something wrong. You've got to come to terms with it – not that you want to. You kid yourself that there isn't anything wrong but you see the person realises it themselves ...

'His personality changed completely. He lost interest in everything – just wanted to sit, didn't want to speak or see anyone, or expect me to either. Instead of his cheerful and very polite self (he was always a gentleman) I never knew what he was going to say to people and friends.

'The doctor made him retire at the age of 56 on medical grounds. He didn't want to go out and didn't want me to either. I felt like a caged animal. He didn't like the television or radio on, wouldn't read books or the newspaper, and suddenly didn't like me doing it either – even sitting quietly doing a crossword would annoy him. So I ended up living on my nerves and had to go to the doctor myself. I needed treatment myself, but it helped when the doctor explained to me that it was the dementia that was making my husband behave like this. I thought our marriage was on the rocks.'

What is dementia?

Although the diseases which cause dementia are more common in older people, dementia is not part of the normal ageing process. Whereas mild forgetfulness may be a part of growing older, the severe memory loss which characterises dementia is not. There are some rare illnesses which can cause dementia in people as young as 35.

The term dementia describes a group of symptoms which result from the destruction of brain cells. Although dementia is a physical illness, most of the symptoms and problems caused by the illness require psychiatric expertise and care. Dementia gradually affects the ability of people affected to:

- remember things for more than a few seconds;
- make sense of the world around them;
- cope with the tasks of daily living;
- express their feelings;
- take initiatives or make plans;
- think clearly and solve problems;
- cope with an over-stimulating environment;
- behave in the normal ways they have learned during their lives.

Common symptoms

No two people with dementia are alike and different people may develop different symptoms, depending upon their personality and the illness that has caused the dementia. The most common problems are:

Memory loss This is often an early sign that something is amiss, and may at first be indistinguishable from forgetfulness brought on by being under stress or feeling depressed. As time goes on, there may be times when your relative is confused about where she is, and she may wander away from home and forget the way back.

Changes in personality People who are struggling to function with a progressively limited thinking capacity may over-react to everyday situations and tasks. Previously mild-mannered people may become abusive or aggressive. Some people lose all social inhibitions and behave in ways that would have been outrageous to them before they were ill. Some people start to swear when they have never used such language before. Others become sweet-natured and passive. Changes in behaviour are caused by damage to the brain and are not something the person can control or prevent.

Difficulty in communicating The person with dementia may have problems in making herself understood – for example forgetting the names of familiar objects or people. She may also have difficulty in understanding what is said to her and may be unable to act on instructions. An explanation that she has previously understood may be forgotten a few minutes later. This is often misunderstood as uncooperative behaviour, but it is not something that the person is doing intentionally.

Loss of practical skills Simple tasks like unbuttoning a shirt can become impossible. Daily activities such as feeding, dressing and washing may become more difficult as the illness becomes worse.

The person with dementia has no control over these changes: they are directly due to damage to the brain.

Most forms of dementia are irreversible. Although physical treatment is limited, much can be done to help the person with dementia manage the illness and to help the family to plan for the future. For this reason, it is essential that your relative is under the care of a sympathetic family doctor.

Ruling out other causes of the symptoms

One of the reasons it is essential to consult a doctor and to get a proper medical diagnosis is that there may be other reasons for the symptoms which *can* be treated.

- Some physical infections, particularly chest and urinary infections, may interfere with the normal functioning of the brain. Treating the infection – or withdrawing the drugs that are being used – may return the person to normal again.
- Thyroid gland deficiency and vitamin deficiencies may also affect the functioning of the brain, causing confusion, but they can be cured with treatment.
- A combination of drugs and alcohol can make a person confused, as can a high dosage of a prescribed drug. Adjusting the dosage of a common drug such as sleeping tablets may make the symptoms disappear.
- Brain tumours or head injuries can affect the brain and may respond to treatment.
- Some life changes such as bereavement or a sudden shock may be associated with a period of confusion. Sometimes this is because the person has become depressed. Severe depression may appear to be the same as dementia: the depressed person may feel so low that she forgets to eat, neglects her hygiene

and appears confused and unable to answer simple questions. With proper care and treatment, these symptoms can be reversed – depression is treatable.

Illnesses that cause dementia

Alzheimer's disease

You may have been told that your relative probably has 'Alzheimer's disease' or a 'dementia of the Alzheimer type'. The vagueness of the description is because a definite diagnosis can be confirmed only by brain biopsy (examination of tissue removed from the brain) or upon examining the brain after death.

Alzheimer's disease is the most common cause of dementia. It is usually a disease of old age, but occasionally it affects people in middle age. It may affect men or women, regardless of their class, race or intellectual ability.

Alzheimer's is a progressive physical disease which causes a decline in the ability to remember, to learn, to think and to reason. As yet there is no specific medical treatment or cure available. Medical specialists tend to concentrate more on attempting to alleviate the consequences of the condition.

Scientists are still trying to find out what causes the illness. They know that changes take place within the brain which cause the abnormal functioning of brain cells. Under a microscope, changes in the structure of the brain can be seen: these changes are known as tangles and plaques. The tangles consist of fibrillary protein abnormalities within brain cells. The plaques are associated with deposits of another abnormal protein, which cause a gradual decline in the ability to learn, reason and remember.

Recent research has identified a genetic cause in a small number of families, and many people who have Down's syndrome unfortunately develop Alzheimer's in middle age. But the majority of cases of Alzheimer's disease are not hereditary.

Our lack of real knowledge about the causes of the illness have led to a number of commonly held myths. The following are some of the factors that we know do *not* cause Alzheimer's disease:

■   underuse or overuse of the brain;
■   infection: Alzheimer's cannot be 'caught';
■   stress, bereavement, retirement or other major life changes: symptoms may become more obvious, but they were probably present (albeit well disguised) before the event;
■   hardening of the arteries.

There has been some circumstantial evidence linking aluminium with Alzheimer's disease. However, since the majority of elderly people do *not* get Alzheimer's disease despite the widespread presence of aluminium in the environment, researchers do not suggest that aluminium alone is a cause of Alzheimer's.

Multi-infarct dementia

This is the second most common type of dementia. The person suffers a series of small strokes which destroy small areas of the brain. 'Infarction' means the death of brain tissue. This happens when small blood vessels in the brain burst, or are blocked by blood clots. This damage can lead to dementia. Sometimes Alzheimer's disease and multi-infarct dementia occur together.

Multi-infarct dementia may start suddenly, and the small strokes can lead to a sudden decline followed by a stabilising period until the next stroke.

Joyce

'My mother had multi-infarct dementia and she'd be fine for a while, then she'd have a mini-stroke. Although her speech was still there, maybe her hand wouldn't work and then maybe a bit of memory would go – or then she'd fall out of bed in the night and stay there until next day. Then a week later she'd be fine – back to normal again. Then she'd go on for two or three months, then it would all start again.'

Sometimes further strokes can be prevented and the dementia halted; in other cases the progression cannot be stopped.

Other types of dementia

A number of more rare conditions can also cause dementia. Pick's disease particularly affects the front of the person's brain, leading to loss of judgement and inhibitions. An illness related to Parkinson's disease, Lewy body dementia, can follow a different course from Alzheimer's disease, with many spells of confusion, hallucinations and a rapid decline to death.

Huntington's chorea is an inherited degenerative brain disease which is gradually progressive, and dementia occurs in the majority of cases. The first symptoms may be slight twitching of the limbs or muscles of the face.

People suffering from AIDS (acquired immune deficiency syndrome) may also develop dementia in the later stages of the illness. The AIDS virus itself may attack certain types of brain cell, or it may be that people with AIDS develop viral infections of the brain because of their weakened immune system.

For more *i*nformation

🛈 *Caring for the Person with Dementia: A guide for families and other carers* by Chris Lay and Bob Woods, published by the Alzheimer's Disease Society (address on p 109).

🛈 Alzheimer's Disease Society Information Sheet 1 *Alzheimer's disease – What is it?*

🛈 *Understanding Dementia*, a free booklet available from MIND Publications (address on p 112).

🛈 *AIDS Dementia*, a free booklet available from AVERT (address on p 109).

Possible stages of dementia

Everyone with dementia will have a different experience of the illness. Although the disease will get progressively worse, there is no way of knowing how rapidly this will happen. Not everyone will suffer all the symptoms mentioned here, but if you want to prepare for the worst it may help to know about how the disease can progress and to anticipate the potentially disabling effects of severe dementia.

Ted

'I returned home to find the entire contents of a door to door salesman's carrier had been purchased.'

'My wife is now at an advanced stage of Alzheimer's disease. I did not fully recognise the condition until about six years ago when there were several crises which left no doubt about the need for a total change of lifestyle. It built up over a year or two. Once, she went to babysit for our grandchildren but came home within an hour. When I asked her why she had come back so soon, she explained that our daughter had said, "You will not be bothered after an hour when they will have gone to sleep." Another time, she was two hours late after taking a circuitous route for what should have been a five-minute car journey.

Further incidents left me in no doubt about her need for care. One day she came home by taxi following the theft of the car. She was interviewed by the police and gave a full report to them about the time and place from which the car was stolen. The car was found outside a shop which my wife had visited in a pedestrian precinct. The police took no action.

'Not long after this my wife, who was renowned for her thrift, bought £80 worth of handmade chocolates for a token present for a child's birthday. Another day, I returned home to find the entire contents of a door-to-door salesman's carrier had been purchased.'

The early stages

It is often hard to say exactly when the disease starts, and it may be only in looking back that you can tell when it began. The person with the illness will probably find ways of covering up mild memory lapses; spouses, friends or work colleagues will often try to 'cover' for embarrassing mistakes or problems which occur. At the time, any difficulties may be put down to increased pressure or stress, or perhaps a change in lifestyle or surroundings. Your relative may:

- repeat conversations;
- have odd moments of appearing puzzled and confused;
- be less adaptable and willing to try new things, becoming increasingly withdrawn;
- over-react to small mistakes;
- deny problems, or blame others for stealing items she has mislaid;
- forget recent events;
- forget dates she has previously remembered, such as birthdays.

John

'As I looked round I saw her put the tea-bags in the kettle, not the tea pot. I said, "Dot, whatever are you doing?" That was over three years ago: I am now her carer, watching over her every hour of the day.'

Those first days of concern are very hard. You are worried, but also probably trying to maintain that everything is normal. You may even feel you are being disloyal to talk about your worries to anyone else. This is understandable – but for both your sake and your relative's, you do need to seek help before the situation reaches a point of crisis. Typical examples of a crisis might be that your relative has a fall or loses her way home or leaves the gas tap on.

If you suspect a person close to you may be developing dementia, you need to:

- consult a doctor as soon as possible to get a proper diagnosis and to make sure that she is not suffering from an illness which can be treated (see pp 4–5);
- find out more about dementia.

The early involvement of a good family doctor can help you to find help and to plan for the future. The GP should help you and your relative by:

- referring your relative for appropriate tests;
- organising treatment and management programmes with other professionals;
- keeping in touch to provide continuing care and supervision.

The dementia progresses

At this stage, it becomes harder for the problems to be disguised. Your relative may:

- often repeat herself and forget the names of people and objects;
- get lost while out walking, especially if she is away from familiar routes;
- leave saucepans to boil dry or the gas unlit;
- confuse day and night – wanting to go out in the middle of the night and sleep all day;
- stop doing normal household tasks such as shopping and cleaning;
- forget to eat, or ask for another meal directly after eating;
- neglect or forget personal hygiene;
- see or hear things that are not there;
- think things have been stolen and accuse their family of stealing them.

Ken

'At first we laughed it off when he got his actions mixed up. Then his personal hygiene began to deteriorate, he had to be reminded to wash and shave and change his clothes. Money would go from his pocket and he would blame us for its disappearance. He would forget events that happened minutes earlier and get mixed up with days of the week. He imagined that I was a member of the Communist Party because I had a red pullover on, and me a practising Catholic. All these events occurred over a six-month period before we began to realise it was something more than just old age.'

The later stages

By this stage, the person with dementia needs constant care and supervision. Your relative may:

- need help with dressing;
- be incontinent;
- need supervision during washing and bathing;
- not be aware of the time of the day, where she lives or the identities of close friends and relatives;
- be confused about her own age and phase of life, asking to speak to people who are dead or wanting to go to work or school;
- have great difficulties with even simple conversation and understanding;
- be constantly restless and prone to wandering, especially at night;
- have fixed ideas – for example looking for people or objects that are not there;
- be verbally abusive or aggressive, especially when feeling under pressure;
- have fits, lose consciousness or make involuntary movements;
- lose weight and have some wasting of the muscles.

Ken

'When they think you're somebody else – that's the worst part. You're not theirs any more and they're not yours. It's a stranger you're looking after and you're probably a stranger to them.'

Looking after someone in the later stages of dementia is a full-time nursing job. Your relative will probably need help with all aspects of her life: you will need to ensure that the home is safe, that she is eating well, being washed, taking exercise and under the supervision of a doctor. In addition to physical care, your relative will need to feel secure and loved. This is a tall order for one person (or even for families sharing the care) to take on; the demands of such care can place severe restrictions on a carer's life and strains on their own health.

Getting medical help

Getting a diagnosis of dementia is not always a straightforward matter. In the early stages, it may be difficult to identify an illness, particularly if the person is making an effort to disguise or deny the problems she is having.

Edwin

'My wife was getting steadily worse and I tried to get her to see the doctor, but she wouldn't go. I consulted our doctor and explained the position to him. He said that's okay, leave it to me. By this time, my wife was beginning to realise something was wrong. Anyway the doctor duly arrived a few days later and made the excuse that while he was in the area, never having visited the house before, he had decided to call in. After a while he managed to persuade my wife to go into the hospital for tests, to which she reluctantly agreed.'

Kit

'Summing up my feelings and experiences of caring, I would say to others, first and foremost, seek the help of a doctor as soon as things start to go wrong. Then try to get some respite care.'

Consulting the GP

Here are some tips if your relative or friend is reluctant to consult the GP (general practitioner or family doctor):

■ First, discuss the matter with her and try to identify the reason behind the reluctance. Does she really believe there is nothing wrong with her? Or is she frightened that something is the matter and hoping that it will just go away again?

■ If it is your partner you are worried about, you could suggest that both of you visit the GP for a routine health check.

■ Speak to the GP yourself and explain your concerns and try to enlist his or her help. The GP may be able to arrange a home visit or have other ideas about how to deal with the problem tactfully.

■ If the GP is unable to help, you could try your local psychiatric service, which may be able to arrange for a community psychiatric nurse to pay a visit (see p 44).

Once you have succeeded in arranging a visit to the GP, here are some points to bear in mind:

■ Do not underplay your concern: remember you are not being disloyal in bringing the difficulties out into the open. Any symptoms are not your relative's fault and you need to feel able to talk frankly about your worries.

■ If you think your relative is going to deny having any difficulties, you may need to make an appointment to see the GP on your own. If you do this, book the appointment in your relative's name so that the doctor will have her notes to hand.

■ Before you go, draw up a list of what you want to say about symptoms that are worrying you, and note down any questions you have.

■ Ask for further explanation if the doctor uses words or expressions you do not understand.

Once the GP has ruled out other possibilities and considers your relative may have some form of dementia, there are a number of questions you will probably want to address to the doctor immediately, such as:

- Is the dementia caused by an illness that can be treated?
- How will the dementia develop and what symptoms can be expected?
- How long is your relative going to be able to live in her own home?

However well-trained your GP is, he or she will not be able to give you definite answers to these questions because there is still so much to be learnt about the causes and treatment of dementia and because everyone with dementia experiences the illness in a different way. Your GP can give you his or her informed judgement but cannot predict what will happen. There are questions to which you should receive full answers, however:

- What treatment will be offered and how will it help?
- What support will be offered to the family and/or other carers?

The GP should wait for the results of a further assessment by a consultant before giving full medical advice. If your relative is not offered a more comprehensive medical assessment by a consultant specialist, you can ask whether this might be appropriate.

Referral to a specialist

Depending on your relative's age and symptoms, she may be referred to any of the consultant specialists below.

If your relative is below retirement age, she may be referred to a **psychiatrist**, a specialist in problems to do with mental health, or a **neurologist**, someone who specialises in disorders of the brain and nervous system.

People over retirement age will probably see a **psychogeriatrician**, who is a psychiatrist with further training in the mental health problems of older people. The psychogeriatrician will spot any physical complications and may refer your relative for more help to a **geriatrician**, who specialises in illnesses and disabilities in older people.

Consultants often prefer to assess people in their own home. They may also want to talk to you or another close relative or friend. At this stage, the consultant will still be looking for other causes for the apparent dementia, in case there are problems that can be treated.

Further physical and mental tests may be needed; sometimes this could mean a short stay in hospital or a visit to a local day hospital.

During the visit, your relative may be given:

- blood tests;
- a very thorough physical examination;
- a number of tests to assess reasoning and memory;
- a CAT (computerised axial tomography) scan – a sophisticated X-ray of the brain.

If a diagnosis of dementia is made, the consultant should tell you as the carer and give you some general idea of what to expect in the future. A major issue both for you and for the consultant is how much you tell your relative. The issues involved here are discussed on pages 17–20.

Often the consultant will be one of a team of professionals. Others in the team may include a **clinical psychologist**, who specialises in the study of human and animal behaviour (psychology) and is also trained in health problems, **community psychiatric nurses** (see p 44), **social workers** (see p 47) and **occupational thera-pists** (see p 45).

Further assessment by the team should determine your relative's capabilities and needs and identify what support should be offered. An appropriate treatment care plan should be offered, which might include, for example:

- advice on medication;
- respite care at a local day centre;
- regular visits from a community psychiatric nurse.

Reactions to the diagnosis

How you feel when you hear the diagnosis of dementia will vary according to how you are told and whether you suspected this was the problem. Any of the following reactions are quite usual.

Shock and a feeling of numbness You – and your relative if she has been told of the diagnosis – may feel suddenly alone and cut off from the rest of the world. Although the doctor and others may have given you information about what the diagnosis means, you may find you can't remember a word of what they have said.

Relief It may feel like a huge weight has been lifted to realise that the strange behaviour of someone you care for is the result of a physical illness rather than a problem in your relationship. If your relative has been denying that she has any problems, it may be a confirmation that you were right and not after all going crazy yourself.

Panic As the news sinks in, you may feel frightened and confused and not know where to turn. You will probably have a great many questions that need answers and – particularly if you have other family responsibilities – you may be unsure about how much practical caring you will be willing or able to offer when your relative becomes more ill.

Anger and a feeling of loss You may feel angry at the injustice of it all, and grief at the loss of the person you once knew. These feelings may recur over the period that the person you care for continues to suffer the illness. You can read more about this in Chapter 6 (see pp 95–105).

For more help and advice

i Contact the national association that represents people with the illness your relative has been diagnosed as having, for example the **Alzheimer's Disease Society** (address on p 109). They will give you information about the illness and advice on how to manage; they will also put you in touch with local groups.

i Contact the **Carers National Association** (address on p 110). They will listen to your feelings, fears or worries and put you in touch with a local group or contact.

i Find out about local carers' groups or organisations that provide advice and support. Your local **Council for Voluntary Service**, **Age Concern** organisation or **reference library** (all will be listed in the telephone directory) should be able to point you in the right direction.

What should you tell your relative?

Does your relative know what is happening to her?

Tom

'In the early stages, my wife would say, "Heavens – whatever is the matter with me?" when she couldn't get a word out. She knew what she wanted to say but she couldn't find the word.'

Songul

'She would tap her head and say, "Oh dear, my brain's not working properly." She was aware that she was not retaining information for any length of time.'

The degree of self-awareness may depend on which part of the brain has been damaged. There is some evidence that people with multi-infarct dementia retain more insight because damage to the brain is patchy. If your relative is aware of her difficulties, she may be living in dread of making a fool of herself and is probably worried about failing at simple tasks. Frustration and fear may be expressed in bouts of uncharacteristic anger or aggression.

In the early stages of dementia your relative may not yet be very ill, but it can be a particularly stressful time for the person who is looking after her. You may feel very protective and try to hide the severity of the problems. You may tolerate abusive behaviour or an uncharacteristic mess in the house to avoid upsetting her. Preserving her self-esteem and dignity may be more important to you. As the person with dementia becomes less aware of what is happening, it becomes easier for the carer to accept help from outside.

Although it is hard to know how much a person in the later stages of dementia does understand, carers often believe that some awareness is retained, even if it is only momentary. People with dementia may also preserve some accurate memories of the past and often respond to expressions of caring and affection.

George

'On the day that she died she "came to" when I went to see her in hospital. As God is my judge, she said to me, 'You have been a good son to me and I want you to give me a hug and kiss before you go home." I will treasure that memory for the rest of my life.'

On hearing the diagnosis

Should a person with dementia be informed about their diagnosis? This is a dilemma which has no simple answer and still divides the medical profession. Some argue that the information would be too difficult to handle and could lead to depression and further difficulties. Another view is that people have a right to know what is wrong with them so that they can make informed choices about their life.

What consultants tell their patients

A survey reported by the Alzheimer's Disease Society showed that the majority of psychiatrists who answered the questionnaire rarely told their patients of their diagnosis. However, the approach to patients with mild dementia showed considerable variation in practice, with a slight majority in favour of disclosing the diagnosis. With patients who had severe dementia, nearly all the carers were told but few of the patients.

The reasons doctors give for not telling their patients the diagnosis is that with severe dementia they believe people are incapable of absorbing the information, and with mild dementia the diagnosis is still too uncertain. Some say that patients should be told only if they ask to be. Another approach is to avoid the term 'dementia' and to use alternatives like 'failure of brain cells', 'memory problems' and 'brain shrinkage'. Others in the survey merely said they were 'economical with the truth'.

What carers tell the people they care for

The Alzheimer's Disease Society reports that carers appear to agree with this practice. But it places the carer in a difficult position: what do you do if you are told that your relative has Alzheimer's disease or is suffering from some other form of dementia? Do you tell the person what you know?

The answer will always be a personal choice. It has to depend on your knowledge of your relative. If she is denying that there is anything wrong, it will probably only distress her further to try to explain that she is ill. You also need to take into account her past feelings about mental illness and dementia.

However, if she is aware that something is wrong and asking what is happening, you do have to address the question. Some people prefer to know what is happening so that they can understand that there is physical cause for the strange lapses they are experiencing. It may also make it easier for them to accept that they do need help in managing the condition.

How you explain what is happening is a sensitive issue which only you can judge. Some people are able to accept a straightforward explanation and are lucid enough to understand what they're being told. More often, though, carers adopt a more gentle approach, similar to that of the psychiatrists in the survey, saying something like 'You have a memory problem'.

The consultant, GP or community psychiatric nurse should be able to advise you and to help you talk to your relative. It is important that some understanding is reached because your relative needs to know that you, as the carer, will sometimes need a break.

The right to be consulted

Whether or not you choose to tell your relative the bald truth about her condition, there are many ways in which you can involve your

19

relative in managing her illness. When she is only mildly affected she may be able to work with you to devise memory aids and methods of keeping the day-to-day routine going. At the early stage of the illness, it may be helpful for you both to share your sadness and concerns about the future. Counselling may also be useful for your relative in coming to terms with the new situation and accepting the limitations the illness imposes on her.

Even as the illness progresses and you are unsure about how much your relative understands, remember to keep talking to her: tell her what you are doing and why, and continue to let her feel that she has a part in deciding things herself. Try not to talk about her in her presence, and ask others to do the same.

For more *i*nformation

i Alzheimer's Disease Society booklet *Facing Dementia: Useful information for people with dementia* and Advice Sheet No 19 *What if I have dementia?*

2 Thinking ahead

You know that your relative, partner or friend has an illness which causes dementia. What do you do now? How can you help your relative remain independent as long as possible? Where should he live? Who needs to be told about the disease? If you are still reeling under the shock and wondering how to cope, this is not a time for making hasty decisions. There are important decisions to be made, but you need time to talk over alternatives with other members of the family and – if the dementia is not too far advanced – with your relative himself.

This chapter will help you to think through some of the options and to consider some of the difficult decisions you are facing. Essentially, the aim is to prevent or to minimise a crisis in the future.

Petra

'One night she rang and said "I'm on fire"'

'My mother has had multi-infarct dementia since undergoing bypass surgery when she was 78. She came through the operation very successfully with no further angina. She also appeared to get over the confusional state. However, over the years she had many mini-strokes and she gradually "changed" mentally. The GP just dismissed it, but when you are close to someone you know they are changing.

'Later on she would ring us up at night (she lived alone) – sometimes twice. I would try and talk her into going back to bed, but she couldn't remember where it was – although saying "the pink bedroom" was sometimes enough. She wouldn't remember the next day having rung.

'One night she rang and said, "I'm on fire." Although there was no open fire I thought, supposing this was true – somehow she had caught her clothing alight. I dressed and went to see her (it was 4.30 am).

'When I arrived, not knowing what I would find, she came to the door – nothing wrong! When I queried this, she said, "I felt as though I was on fire."

'I became so tired with frequent phone calls at night and then going to work next day. Although I only worked part time, I still found that, with all the worry, it was too much and I decided to take early retirement.

'By this time my mother slept in the chair all night and was creating a fuss about changing her clothes. One day, when my car was in dock, my mother rang not knowing where she was and feeling very frightened. I rang the student social worker who said she would visit – and did immediately. She stayed an hour trying to calm my mother down. I have never been so grateful.'

Staying independent

If your relative wishes to continue living in his own home, it is important to minimise the risks of doing so. But it is impossible to take away all risk without forfeiting the person's own dignity and independence.

Where the person with dementia is living with a partner, it is sometimes the case that the person caring prolongs the *notion* of independence long after the ill person has in fact become quite dependent. The appearance of normality is often the most important thing, but at some cost to the carer.

Where the person with dementia lives alone, the level of risk that is acceptable can often be a contentious issue between different family members and may require some open discussion. Family members need to explore why they hold different views: there may be misunderstandings, unrealistic assumptions or unnecessary fears.

In an ideal situation, family members work out together at an early stage how they will help their relative. This may be through regular visits or an agreement to take the person out once a week. Others who live further away may help with care costs or give the main carer a break while he or she takes a holiday.

If these negotiations are difficult, it may help to have an impartial third party who can help the discussion along – a social worker or community psychiatric nurse may be willing to help.

Cutting down the risk

Susan

'My mother had a fire cooking a chop. She fell asleep, so setting the chop on fire. I don't really know how she got out, but it took my husband and me 15 hours to wash down the walls and ceilings and then another morning to repaint the ceilings. Since then, the cooker has been disconnected and meals on wheels organised. I or my aunty provide other meals.'

Whether your relative is living with you or in his own home, there are a number of measures you can take to minimise risks:

Medicines and poisons Lock away any cleaning fluids or other poisonous household substances and make sure you or a visiting nurse supervises any medication.

Fire If your relative smokes, there is a real risk of fire. If you do not wish to persuade him to stop, make sure smoke detectors are fitted to the home. Any fire or heater should have a fire guard.

Gas If your relative is prone to turning on the gas and leaving the cooker unlit, you may have to consider having the gas turned off and arranging for meals to be brought into the home. You can also fit a gas detector in the kitchen, if someone is visiting regularly.

Falls Check the house for dangerous surfaces – slippery floors, loose carpets and so on. Ask the occupational therapist or social worker (see p 45) for advice about aids such as a bath seat or mat to prevent slipping and handrails for the stairs and by the bath and toilet. Make sure the lighting is bright.

Locks You may need to remove locks from interior doors such as bathroom and toilet doors. Keep a set of duplicate front door keys so that you can enter in an emergency.

Warmth Ensure the house is well insulated. If your relative has a low income and is worried about the cost of heating, there may be help available to cover the cost of insulation.

Talk to neighbours Ask friendly neighbours or friends of your relative to keep an eye out for any trouble. Make sure you leave a telephone number where you can be contacted.

Although everyone will have their own view about what risks they feel they can comfortably tolerate, there are some which cannot be ignored. It may often be a point of crisis when something has happened that makes you realise how vulnerable your relative has become.

Eileen

'My mother seemed to be managing quite well on her own and was fiercely independent. She had always been very houseproud and managed to keep the place looking nice. I sometimes worried if she was eating properly, but the social worker arranged for a private agency to bring in a hot meal once a day and I felt happier after that. The crunch came when I discovered she'd paid out hundreds of pounds to have her house double-glazed, but the house already had double glazing and they had fitted it on top of the existing lot.'

For more *i*nformation

i Alzheimer's Disease Society Advice Sheet 4 *Safety in the home*.

i *Safe as Houses*, available from the Alzheimer's Disease Society (address on p 109).

i Age Concern England Factsheet 33 *Feeling safer at home and outside*.

i Age Concern England Factsheet 1 *Help with heating*.

Driving

A car is often the last symbol of independence; for many carers, their relative having to give it up marks a real crisis point. Hard as it is, you may have to point out to your relative that his insurance is unlikely to cover him if he has had a diagnosis of dementia (assuming he is aware of the diagnosis). The risk to your relative in continuing to drive is just as high as if he were losing his sight.

You will have to be firm on this subject and you may need to ask the GP or other members of the family to help you to persuade your relative to stop driving. The Driver and Vehicle Licensing Centre can advise you on the medical aspects of fitness to drive; you (or the GP) can ring them on a special number: 01792 783686.

Try to find some way of compensating for the loss of the car by organising family and friends to be available to offer lifts, and find out if your local council has a scheme for cheap or free public transport for people with disabilities.

Other ways of helping your relative to stay independent

The following are some positive steps you can take to help a person with dementia stay independent as long as possible:

Keep things simple and stick to a routine

If your relative finds a task difficult, try to break it down into smaller bits. Don't offer too many choices at once: two is enough.

When memory is failing, a regular routine will help him to remember what is happening.

Use memory aids

These are aids that can jog the memory or help your relative find his way about, for example:

■ Put labels on the doors of rooms.
■ Make lists of things to do that day, and times that visitors or nurses are expected.
■ Put familiar objects and photos of family and friends on view.
■ Have a calendar on view and a clock with a large, clear face that can be read easily.

Keep communicating

Although your relative may be suffering increasing problems with understanding and expressing himself, don't overlook the possibility that the cause might be something unrelated:

■ Is his hearing impaired, or a hearing aid not working?
■ Are his dentures loose?
■ Is his sight failing? Do his glasses need changing?

In general communication, try to keep sentences simple, and speak clearly and slowly. Don't collude with delusions, but avoid confrontations: gently change the subject or distract him with something else. Don't forget that physical communication may be the best way to get through – a comforting hug or a squeeze of the hand.

Watch his general health and diet

A balanced diet and physical exercise will help keep your relative active as long as possible.

Where should your relative live?

Moving in with you

If you are not living under the same roof, try not to be pressured by others into thinking you must move your relative into your home. This is not necessarily the best solution: familiar surroundings are important for people who are confused and moving may take away any remaining independence. If your relative is used to living alone and wishes to continue to do so there are ways of achieving this (see pp 22–26).

If you do decide that it would be a good idea for your relative to move in with you, you will need to think about:

Your relationship with your relative What was this like before he became ill? If you never got along in health, you are bound to run up against problems in sickness.

Finances What impact will the move have on your income or your relative's? Check with the local advice agency or Citizens Advice Bureau if State pensions or benefits will be affected.

The views of all the people in the household, particularly if space is limited. Does your partner support the move? How do your children feel about it? And how will your relative cope with living alongside children and teenagers?

Planning breaks from caring How will you and your family get time to relax and to get away from the difficulties of looking after someone with dementia?

Chris

'I have had my mother (now aged 94) living with me for 20 years. She has always been demanding so it is difficult to know when dementia began. The hardest thing was to bring up two strong-willed teenagers and cope with Mum, who was then in the early stages of dementia. I'm also a part-time teacher – not exactly a stress-free job. I think we cope in different ways. The children are now married and away from it, having been told by me never to have me living with them. Me – I escape and cope by relaxing with my dogs and by having Mum go to a day centre and into phased care to give me a break.'

Try to involve your relative in the move as much as possible unless he is incapable of understanding what is happening. He may be feeling anxious and suspicious anyway, and attempting to move him without his participation may make it more difficult to get him to settle in the new environment.

Even if your relative comes to live in your home, there may still be a point when residential or nursing home care becomes necessary. Although it may be hard to think about now, you may be able to avoid a crisis in the future if you are realistic about where your own 'cut-off' point will be. If you do not recognise your limits, you are in danger of becoming ill yourself, which may mean the person you care for being admitted to alternative care in an emergency. Everyone has different limits, but some common critical points for carers are when the person with dementia:

- regularly becomes aggressive;
- is frequently incontinent;
- often does not sleep at night;
- regularly does not recognise the carer;
- constantly wanders.

Moving in with your relative

Some people choose to move in with the person who needs to be cared for. Although this may be easier for the person with dementia, it can be a huge step for the carer, involving a great deal of disruption.

> ### *Rose*
>
> 'When it first became apparent that my mother could not live alone in her home, after a heart attack and hospitalisation, which made her even more confused, I had to reorganise my whole life within a week or two so that I could move down to where she lived. I still continued with full-time employment in a demanding job, but I had also to find tenants for my house, organise furniture removal down to my mother's home, arrange for a convalescent home for her till all ends were tied up, and finally buy a newer car to see me through the daily commuting safely. On arriving at my mother's home, where my sister was temporarily holding the fort, my mother looked me squarely in the face and said, "Who are you?"'

You also need to find out what the financial and legal implications could be if you give up your home to move in with your relative. If your relative later becomes too ill to remain at home and needs to move into a care home, your right to stay in the house or flat may be in jeopardy. You should take advice before making any final decision.

For more *i*nformation

 Age Concern England Factsheet 10 *Local authority charging procedures for residential and nursing home care*. This gives detailed information about how the value of your home is treated if you go into a residential or nursing home.

 Age Concern England Factsheet 38 *Treatment of the former home as capital for people in residential and nursing homes*.

Moving together

If you and your relative are already living together but in a house or flat that is difficult to manage, you may consider moving to a flat or retirement home. You need to weigh up whether the benefits of moving will make it worth managing the difficulties of leaving familiar surroundings. Such benefits might be:

■ good support services, perhaps in sheltered accommodation with a warden on call;

■ being closer to friends or family who will help you;

■ a home where the person you look after will be at less risk.

Before you commit yourself to a move, check the financial and legal implications of moving, for example whose name the new property should be under.

T elling other people

Once a diagnosis of dementia has been confirmed, it is vital that other people are informed. You need to think about:

■ how your relative feels about letting others know;

■ who to tell;

■ what you will say;

■ ways they can help.

Telling family and friends

If your relative is still lucid and in the early stages of dementia, he may have strong feelings about letting others know what is happening – assuming, of course, that he is aware that he is ill. Take time to talk it over with your relative and agree who should be told and what should be said. Any resistance on his part may be due to a feeling of shame or embarrassment – reassure him that friends and family will find it easier to help him if they understand what is happening.

If, for any reason, you have chosen to shield your relative from the full truth of the diagnosis, be sure to tell only those people who you can trust to be discreet.

A remarkable account of one woman's decline into dementia – *Living in the Labyrinth* by Diana Friel McGowin – describes the experience of living with the disease. She describes how she tried to hide her illness and why she felt unable to share her worries:

'I considered Dr T's repeated instructions to have a family confer-
ence and advise my children of my situation. So far, I had not
followed them. I could not bring myself to confide in my children.
I could not even accept it myself. Intellectually, I knew my condition was not cause for shame, yet emotionally I felt ashamed. I was
losing my intelligence, losing my memory, and my directional system was really shot to Hades.

'Embarrassment kept me from confiding in my family and friends.
I had no idea of how they would respond. If they were too conde-
scending and made me feel totally worthless, I would chafe; on the
other hand, if they displayed a "so what" attitude, I would be dev-
astated. It would break my heart.'

Choose a time to talk to family and close friends when you are feeling reasonably calm yourself. They will be understandably upset by
the news and this may be very hard for you.

There is still a lot of misunderstanding about dementia. If it helps,
you could arm yourself with some of the free leaflets produced by
voluntary organisations such as the Alzheimer's Disease Society
(address on p 109). Some relatives may want to deny that there is
anything wrong and you may find it easier to ask the family doctor, social worker or community psychiatric nurse to talk to them.

Doreen

'My husband is in the early stages of dementia and my son just won't
accept it. He keeps telling me it's my fault and I should make sure he's
busy, get him to do some decorating or something instead of sitting in a
chair all day. I've tried to explain what's going on, but he's not really listening. I don't think he wants to see it.'

Telling children

It can be hard to know what to say to children when a grandpar-
ent or other relative is behaving oddly, but they will certainly
understand that something is not right, and shielding children

from the truth is rarely helpful. The best policy is to be as honest as you can and to explain to them what is the matter, in simple language. In addition, they may need some reassurance:

■ Tell them that nothing they have done is to blame for what is happening.

■ Explain that they cannot 'catch' the illness, nor is anyone else in the family likely to get it.

■ Discuss small ways in which they can help and share in your relative's care.

■ Address directly any fears or worries they may have.

They may also need to know what you have told your relative about their condition.

Letting local people know

It may be appropriate to alert other people who live and work nearby – friends, neighbours, local shopkeepers, the milkman and postman. Once they understand that your relative's behaviour is caused by an illness, they may be more sympathetic and willing to keep a watchful eye or help in other ways. You may need to explain that the illness means your relative has difficulty in understanding complex speech and that people should try to speak in short, simple sentences.

Clare

'My husband and I went shopping in town. I parked the car and we went to the library. At this stage, John was still able to cross roads safely. He decided to leave me at the library and go on to the bakers and meet me there. Ten minutes later I followed and spent half an hour looking for him, going into all the shops we used. Finally I went back to the car and drove home and he was there. There was no point in getting angry, but following that experience I wrote his address and phone number on a piece of card and put it in his wallet. I also spoke to the shop assistants who knew us. John has speech problems and is unable to communicate with others.'

Looking further ahead

The key to avoiding crises is to plan ahead. If possible, try to plan for the future before the illness has become too serious. You need to:

- find out what help and services are available;
- make sure your relative's finances are in order;
- talk to your relative about his wishes for future care.

Finding out about services

Jim

'My mother had a fear of mental illness. When I first went to visit the day centre, in the early stages of her illness, I knew she would be frightened by the other people there, so I wouldn't let her go there. Now, though, everything has changed. I don't think she notices the odd behaviour of the other people, or maybe in a funny sort of way she feels more at home with people doing silly things like she does. At any rate, she goes there quite happily every day now and it is my lifeline.'

The next chapter tells you how to find out about the practical help that is available. Even if you do not feel ready to use a service now, it is worth finding out what is available: you may feel differently as the illness progresses and your needs, and the needs of your relative, change.

Your relative's finances

Ensure that any financial documents such as mortgage papers, insurance policies and bank statements are easy to find and that all bills are paid up to date.

You can avoid future complications by encouraging your relative to set up an enduring power of attorney (power of attorney in Scotland) while he is still able to understand what is happening and to sign the papers. This means that he appoints someone – or preferably two people – to take over the management of his financial affairs, either immediately or when he is no longer capable of doing so (see pp 81–82 for more details).

Your relative's wishes for future care

One of the most difficult aspects of looking after someone with dementia is having to make decisions on their behalf when they are no longer fit to do so. You may want to enlist the help of the GP, community psychiatric nurse or social worker to talk through some of the decisions that will need to be made in the future. At this stage you may be able to talk to your relative about his own wishes, for example whether he wants to continue living in his own home.

Everyone with a progressive illness like dementia has a different reaction to dealing with the future. Some may deny that anything is wrong, but others may want to ensure that they have a say in their future treatment. If your relative falls into the latter category, it might be a good idea for him to draw up a 'living will' or 'advance directive' while he is still in the early stages of dementia. This is a form of 'anticipated' consent which is drawn up when someone is rational and able to make decisions about the treatment they will or will not receive. In England and Wales, these are now considered to be legally binding as long as the person understood the consequences of the request at the time of making it (see pp 92–93 for details). The position in Scotland is still unclear.

Coping with the responsibility

Ian

'It comes on gradually, you don't take a decision, it just carries on and you find yourself doing it. I remember on one occasion thinking, "Good Lord, if this carries on it won't be her who needs a psychiatrist, it will be me!"'

If you are living with the person you care for, you can find yourself taking on the practical responsibilities of caring without having made a conscious decision to do so. Sons and daughters who live apart from their parents may take a more active decision.

Taking on the practical care of your parent or other relative may not be in the best interests of you, your family or your relative. Hasty decisions are often made in a time of crisis when there is little opportunity to think through the consequences. If you *are* in a position to plan ahead and to make alternative arrangements, ask yourself:

■ Am I the right person to take on the practical care of my relative?
■ How will it affect me and my family in the long term?
■ What are the alternatives?
■ If I do take this on, what help can I count on from other members of the family?

Be realistic about what you can and cannot offer. Taking on the day-to-day care of a person with dementia is both physically and emotionally stressful, and not everybody has a disposition that can cope with the strains that inevitably accompany it. Be assured that there are very few people who can manage to look after a person with dementia without some help.

Your own support

If you do start taking on a caring role, it is vital to set up some regular time away from your relative and make sure you have some emotional support. Everyone has different views on the best way to do this. Here are some options:

Join a carers' group

The particular difficulties of looking after someone with dementia are often best understood by other people who are coping with the same problems. Carers' groups provide an opportunity to offer to and receive support from other people in the same boat. A carers' group may be a general group for people with all kinds of caring responsibilities; a group for those caring for people with a specific illness, such as Alzheimer's disease; or a group for carers of a particular age group or section of the community.

How to find a carers' group

ℹ Ask your local **Council for Voluntary Service**, **Citizens Advice Bureau** or **reference library**.

ℹ Contact your local branch of the **Alzheimer's Disease Society**, **Parkinson's Disease Society** or **Stroke Association**, as appropriate (listed in the telephone directory).

ℹ Ask your **social worker**, **health visitor** or **community psychiatric nurse**.

ℹ Contact the **Carers National Association** head office (address on p 110) for details of local contacts.

Go to a counsellor

Jan

'The psychologist we "talk" to has been an anchor amidst the horrors of the disease, right from three years back, and someone who the children are willing to talk to, knowing their mother is too distressed to listen to their problems.'

If you do not want to join a group, you might want to talk confidentially with a trained counsellor about your worries and frustrations. Although friends and relatives may be able to give you informal support, talking to someone outside the situation can often be a great relief. A counsellor will listen to you and help you to find your own strategies for coping with difficult times.

How to find a counsellor

 Your GP may be able to refer you to a counsellor, but if this is on the NHS, there may be a waiting list.

 If you can afford to pay, you can contact the **British Association for Counselling** (address on p 109) or you could ask the counselling service at the local college or university if they know of people who are freelance counsellors.

Get away from it all

Some people prefer to keep their feelings to themselves. If so, you will still need some outlet – it may be through drawing, writing or physical activity. Whatever your preference, make it a priority and try to ensure that you are able to take a break to make time for this. (See pp 54–57 for information on respite care.)

Caring at a distance

You may not live close to your relative or be the person who is giving the daily care, but there are still things you can do to help: the most important is to support the primary carer. He or she will be taking the brunt of the emotional and physical strain and needs your help.

The following are some ways in which you can offer help:

Keep in touch A regular telephone call or, if possible, regular visits, can help the carer to feel less alone and can help you to get a sense of how the situation is developing.

Gather information The carer may be too distressed, busy or overwhelmed by what is happening to find out about what help is available or to get more information about the illness. Planning ahead is the best way to avoid a crisis: even if the carer is not ready to accept help in the home now, it will help to know where to turn when the time comes.

Recognise the carer's role Carers can often feel like the 'figure in the shadows' when all the attention is on the ill person and his difficulties. Show your appreciation of the work the carer is doing but also make it clear that you do not expect them to carry on beyond their own limits. Be positive and avoid criticism, even if you would do things differently. If you have not spent a long time with your relative, you may not understand how much stress his carer may be under.

Offer help You may not feel able to help with the practical tasks of nursing and caring, but there are probably other tasks which need doing: fixing the car or household appliances, helping sort out the bills, weeding the garden, cooking a meal. If you are not close enough to do these things yourself, can you arrange to pay for someone else to help?

Give the carer a break Even if it is only the odd afternoon trip in the car with your relative, this will give the carer a bit of time off. As the illness progresses, the carer will need longer breaks, so you may want to consider looking after your relative for a weekend or a few days.

May

'My son and daughter-in-law didn't know what to do at first. They all seemed to forget my situation. I have to keep myself active, otherwise I will go down too. My son kept saying, "You should stop at home Mother, do more housework." He's come round now and sees I need to keep up my own life. He takes my husband out for a cup of tea, which is the only time I have the house to myself.'

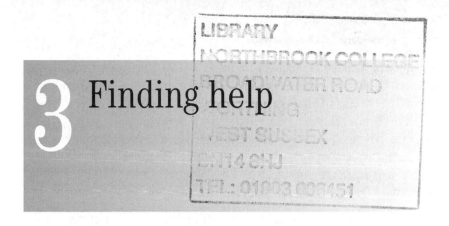

3 Finding help

Looking after a person with dementia is very demanding, and there may come a time when you need to call on others to help. Sometimes a crisis, such as the carer becoming ill, will precipitate this. Sometimes it is the development of new symptoms – such as night wandering – which makes the caring too hard to manage alone.

By finding out what practical services are available and making the system work for you, you can start taking charge of the situation now, before you reach the end of your tether. Even if everything seems manageable at the moment, there will probably come a time when it is not. Contacting people who can help at an early stage in your relative's illness is the best way to avoid a crisis in the future.

This chapter aims to help you find your way around the system.

Ken

'I wish I had known about them earlier and not felt so guilty about asking for help.'

'I have looked after my mother for over 20 years. She was crippled with arthritis and was not able to walk at all well. It is hard to date when the dementia started. In her case it was a slow process. Looking back, I think

39

she must have had it for about six or more years. I first noticed that all was not well in her brain about five years ago. She used to wake me up in the middle of the night (I had installed a bell push on her bedside table and a bell in mine). "There is a waterfall coming down the front of the house," she said. It was not even raining at the time. I told her that there was nothing there. "It's stopped now," she always said. This resulted in many lost nights' sleep. Another cry was that I had my radio on and it was keeping her awake – the radio wasn't on of course.

'Sometimes she would not talk because "they" had installed microphones in the floor and "they" could hear all that was going on in our house. I found it very hard to go out to work – I used to lock her in when I did. I had many years before promised that I would not put her in a home. So I stopped going to work and spent most of my time tending her. I started to get Invalid Care Allowance.

'Things started to get harder. She would not eat unless I was with her and eating. Now and again she would say to me "Who are you?" Once I had an accident on my bicycle and cut my face. She shouted and screamed at me for hours when she saw me. Another time, she attacked me with her walking stick while I was dozing in my chair.

'I was not really coping any more, just surviving. I slept on a camp-bed outside my mother's room because she had started to stumble about during the night. My sister came to stay with us one weekend and my mother was particularly disturbed. She came downstairs and found me, a man of 50 plus, crying and feeling sorry for myself. The next morning she said she was going to take the dog for a walk. She went as far as the village public telephone and phoned the doctor. The result was that we started to get some help.

'Mum goes to a day centre every day now and she has phased care in a care home – two weeks and six weeks at a time on a regular basis. The care workers are wonderful and help me keep my sanity. They tell me all about what is available to help. I wish I had known about them earlier and not felt so guilty about asking for help. It would have saved me so much stress and heartache.'

Who can help?

Services for carers and for people with dementia are not the same in every part of the country. Some places are well served, other areas are lacking in essential services. Some professionals work together as a team, and information you give to one will be passed on, in confidence, to others who can help. Others do not communicate well with each other, and you may find you are telling the same thing to several different people before you get what you want. So be prepared to be persistent, confident in the knowledge that it is your right to receive help to care for your relative. Think ahead about what you may need as the illness progresses and start to put things in motion as soon as possible.

Dealing with professionals

People who work in the health service and social services are there to help you. Remember that you are entitled to:

■ respect for your way of life;
■ choice about how you and your relative wish to live;
■ information about what help is available and how to get it.

You may be under a lot of stress and feeling angry or upset at the situation you find yourself in. This is not an easy time to remain polite but firm. If you do feel nervous dealing with professionals, or you think you might 'lose your cool', ask a friend or relative to be present to back you up. If you think you may forget important information, take notes of what the person says to you, or ask him or her to write it down. Keep a record of dates and times of meetings, so that you can refer back if you do not eventually get what you want. If you have telephone conversations, you can write to the person you spoke to to confirm the content of the call.

There are various people and organisations you can go to for help:

■ the health service (see pp 42–45);
■ social services (see p 46–53);
■ voluntary and private organisations (see p 57).

The McDonald Family

'We care for my wife's older brother (aged 79) who suffers from dementia. He was diagnosed as suffering from Alzheimer's. We must admit to being confused and at times short-tempered, but the very constructive help we received from our GP, district nurses, family and friends and our local branch of Alzheimer Scotland – Action on Dementia helped us to understand and cope with this terrible affliction. Our advice is, if you have any doubts, contact your GP and phone your nearest Alzheimer group.'

Talk to neighbours and friends: since services vary from one area to another, word of mouth is often an important way of finding out what help is available.

Health professionals who can help

The GP

A good relationship with the family doctor is very important both for you and for the person who has dementia. Although there is no treatment at present that can actually reverse or stop the disease, there is a great deal that needs to be done to maintain the affected person's quality of life and to make the problems easier for you (or other carers) to handle.

If you or your relative is not satisfied with the GP, your relative can choose to change doctors. Sometimes you can see a different doctor at the same surgery, without going through the process of changing doctors, if it is a group practice with more than one GP.

Changing your GP

If you want to change doctors you simply find a new doctor in the area who is willing to accept you or your relative on to their list of patients. Contact your local Community Health Council (Health Council in Scotland) or the Health Authority to get names and addresses of GP practices in the area. The Health Authority may be able to tell you if there are any doctors locally who have a special interest in dementia.

Note In 1996, former Family Health Services Authorities and District Health Authorities merged to form new integrated authorities, known as 'Health Authorities'. Regional Health Authorities were abolished at the same time.

There is no need to give a reason for wishing to change doctor either to the new GP or to the previous GP, and you do not need to get the medical card signed by the previous GP.

Once you have been accepted by a new GP practice, your notes should automatically be transferred. When you sign on at a new GP practice, you should take your medical card with you if you have it, but this is not essential.

For more help and advice

ⓘ If you are having difficulty in finding a doctor to take on your relative, the **Health Authority** is responsible for making sure that everyone is registered with a GP.

ⓘ **Your local support or self-help group** for people with your relative's illness may be able to give you names of sympathetic doctors.

ⓘ **Your local Community Health Council (CHC)** can give you advice or information about local health services. If you wish to make a complaint about a doctor and you have been unable to sort the matter out with the doctor concerned, the CHC can advise you about how to make a formal complaint. You can find their address at the local Citizens Advice Bureau or in the telephone directory. In Scotland NHS users are represented by local Health Councils and in Northern Ireland by District Committees.

ⓘ **The NHS Health Helpline** is a freephone information line, established under the Patient's Charter. The number puts you through to a regional office which holds a database on national and local self-help groups. It can provide confidential information on common diseases and conditions, NHS services, waiting times, local Patient's Charter standards, how to make a complaint, and how to maintain good health. Freephone 0800 66 55 44 between 10 am and 5 pm, Monday to Friday.

43

Other health professionals

Geoff

'From the start, the male nurse made it quite clear that they were visiting the two of us and looking at my ability to cope with the situation as well as assessing my wife.'

Community psychiatric nurses (CPNs) are specially trained nurses who help people with mental health problems and their families in the community. They are trained to help people with dementia, but they also offer help and support to people who are caring for those with dementia. Many carers feel their own mental health suffers through the stress of caring for someone with dementia – and the CPN is there to help. The CPN does not usually carry out physical nursing tasks.

How to contact Depending on where you live, you may need a referral from your relative's GP or consultant or you may be able to contact a CPN direct. Your Community Health Council (England and Wales), Local Health Council (Scotland) or District Committee (Northern Ireland) can advise you on how to find a CPN. Some CPNs work from local hospitals. Others are based at GPs' surgeries or community mental health centres.

District nurses are qualified nurses who are further trained in looking after people in their own homes. They can advise on day-to-day care and will perform practical nursing tasks such as changing dressings, giving injections, helping with toileting, etc. They can also give advice about incontinence aids and getting other help.

How to contact Visits can usually be arranged through the GP. You may also be able to contact the district nurse direct through the surgery or health centre.

Health visitors are qualified nurses who are further trained to advise people on health care in their own homes with the aim of anticipating and preventing new health problems. Most health visitors work with people with young children, but a few specialise in working with older people. They do not carry out practical nursing tasks, but they may suggest ways of keeping your relative fit and help to arrange for other support and services.

How to contact You can usually contact the health visitor through the GP or local health centre.

Continence advisers are specially trained nurses who can give advice on toileting problems and continence aids, such as commodes and incontinence pads.

How to contact The adviser often works through the local district nursing team (see above). The Continence Foundation (address on p 110) can give you details about your area. There may also be an incontinence laundry service in your area – ask the social worker, district nurse or health visitor.

Occupational therapists (OTs) can advise about aids and adaptations to the home to maintain your relative's independence as long as possible.

How to contact Depending on the area where you live, you may need to contact health or social services – OTs are employed by both. Ask your GP or social worker.

Chiropodists provide foot care, which is very important in maintaining mobility in older people. The service is available through the NHS for women over 60 and men over 65.

How to contact Ask your GP or health centre for a referral to the district chiropodist. You can also choose to see a chiropodist privately. The letters SRCh after their name mean that they are State registered. There are no regulations governing non-State registered practitioners, so you should enquire about their training.

Counsellors are not usually medically qualified but they are trained to help you to talk, in confidence, about your problems and feelings. Either you or your relative might find it helpful to see a counsellor.

How to contact Many are in private practice, but some GPs now have qualified counsellors attached to their clinic who you can see as an NHS patient.

Note Since April 1996, Health Authorities have had to publish and operate policies, plans and eligibility criteria for a range of NHS continuing health care services, including rehabilitation, respite health care, specialist equipment and continuing inpatient care. Further details are contained in Age-Concern England Factsheet 37 *Hospital discharge arrangements and NHS continuing health care services.*

Approaching social services

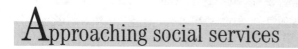

Many services are available under the 1990 NHS and Community Care Act. The key to getting them is to ensure that your relative's needs are assessed by the social services department (known as social work departments in Scotland and the Health and Social Services Board in Northern Ireland). It is well worth getting an assessment at an early stage: the earlier services are arranged, the easier you will find the whole course of the illness.

Under the Carers (Recognition and Services) Act 1995, which came into effect in April 1996, if you are providing a substantial amount of care to your relative on a regular basis, you have the right to ask the local authority to also consider your needs when they are assessing the needs of your relative.

Why involve social services?

If you have had no cause to contact the social services department before, you may be worried about doing so now. Below are some of the reasons why people do not contact social services.

'My relative has enough money to pay for her own help'

You are entitled to use social services, whatever your income. However, unlike with health services, your relative may be asked to make a contribution to some services. As the carer, you should not be asked to pay anything unless you are responsible for the money of the person you care for. Even if your relative has money to pay for care, it is still worth arranging an assessment. The advantage of getting into the 'system' is that the person who assesses your relative may know about all kinds of services that can help you and your relative.

'We want to make our own decisions, not be dictated to by an outsider'

Some people are worried that a social worker may interfere or put their relative into a care home. Social workers have no powers to remove the person you care for or to place her in a home against the wishes of you and your relative except in very limited circum- stances.

On the contrary, they are obliged to work in consultation with you and your relative and should also take your wishes as the carer into account.

'We don't want handouts, we want to be independent'

Social services are not charity: community care services are services provided by the local council for the community it serves. Social services departments are sometimes confused with the Department of Social Security (DSS). The DSS is responsible for welfare benefits; social workers can advise you about your entitlement to benefits but are not employed by the DSS.

How can a social worker help?

Social workers should know what resources and services are available in your community. They should be trained in assessing your situation and the needs of the person you care for. They may also be able to offer practical counselling and to help you and your family to resolve disagreements about the care of your relative. Some social workers specialise in the care of older people.

Getting an assessment

Jane

'The social worker helped me to decide what help we needed and there was no problem when the lady came to give my husband a shower twice a week and dress him afterwards.'

The person you care for may be eligible for a range of different services, some of which you may not even know about. Services that you and your relative might be eligible for include:

- someone to help with cooking, shopping or daily tasks like dressing;
- cooked meals brought into the home;
- sitting services, day centre care or a short stay in a care home to give the carer a break from caring (for information on 'respite care' see pp 54–57);
- aids and equipment to help your relative live as independently as possible;
- counselling (professional help with dealing with the feelings that the illness and the caring situation evoke);
- mobility training for the carer (for example being shown how to lift the person you care for);
- a place in a residential or nursing home.

The person who visits to make the assessment may be a specially trained assessor or someone like a social worker or occupational therapist; they may be called a 'care manager', a 'care coordinator' or a 'community care assessor' – it varies from one area to another. You can expect a lot of form-filling, and very often the person making the assessment will want to visit more than once to get to know you and your relative.

It is important to ask for anything you feel you and your relative need – do not tailor your needs to what you think might be offered.

Try completing some of the following sentences now, thinking separately of your needs and those of the person you care for. If it is still possible, and it feels right, sit down together and discuss your answers.

The thing I would most like is: _____

_____

The most difficult time of the day/night is: _____

_____

What I fear most about the future is: _____

_____

My most difficult problem is: _____

_____

What I miss most is: _____

_____

Although the assessment will be primarily about the needs of the person you care for, the person doing the assessment should also take into account your needs and how much care you are able or willing to give.

The questions asked at your relative's assessment interview will probably cover:

Personal details Name, address, doctor, relationship with carer, housing, etc.

Health details Nature of health problems and the kind of help that is needed with daily living; when and how often help is needed.

What kind of help is already in place, who arranges these services and how much help is given, including what help the carer gives.

What help your relative needs to alleviate physical difficulties, emotional difficulties, lack of social contact, etc.

What help the carer needs in order to continue.

Financial details What income, including benefits, and savings your relative has.

If, during the assessment, social services find that your relative also has health or housing needs, then they should contact the relevant organisations.

Once your relative's needs and your own needs have been identified, the social services department will decide what help, if any, they can offer. If they can offer help, they may put together what is called, in the current jargon, a 'care plan' or 'package of care'.

This is information about the type of help or service they will organise (eg cleaning), how often it will be arranged (eg twice a week) and who will actually provide the service. Local authorities may use their own staff, such as home care workers, or they may arrange for the service to be provided by a voluntary organisation (such as a local Age Concern group) or a private agency. However, the social services department remain responsible for making sure that the services work for your relative.

The sort of help the social services department offers will depend on the needs of you and your relative and on the social services department's own eligibility criteria for getting services.

The care package offered should be tailor-made to make sure the services offered meet the needs which have been identified in the assessment. If you or your relative feel that your needs are not being met, you can make a complaint, as explained on pages 52–54.

Your relative may be asked to make some contribution towards the cost of services, depending on her income and savings. Each local authority sets its own rates for charging for services to help people stay living at home or with a relative, but these must be 'reasonable' for your relative to pay. If the charge is not 'reasonable' you can ask the local authority to reduce or waive the charges. You can also use the local authority's complaints procedure.

Joan lives on her own and is supported by her daughter, who lives in the same town. Social services have arranged for her to have seven days a week private day care, for which Joan contributes £1.85 per day. In addition, someone from a private nursing agency visits every night and helps her to prepare for bed and gives Joan her medication.

Winston also lives on his own. Although his son and daughter-in-law live in the same block of flats, they both work full time. Social services have arranged for someone from a voluntary agency to go in every morning to check his medication and at lunchtime to prepare a meal. Winston contributes £17 a week for this service.

Patricia lives with her husband and also receives private day care throughout the week. A private agency supplies a helper to sleep over at least one night a week to enable her husband to get a night's rest. Social services meet the cost as Patricia and her husband are on a very low income.

Your relative – or you if you are acting on her behalf – should be given a copy of the care plan. You should also ask for a copy of the completed assessment form if you or your relative is not sent one. The care plan should say something about how often the situation will be reviewed and should name the person who is responsible for coordinating the care. The coordinator should also contact health or housing authorities if appropriate.

Note **Since March 1997, local authorities can take their own resources into account when deciding whether someone has a need for a service under the Chronically Sick and Disabled Persons Act 1970, and which services they will then arrange or provide. Services cannot be withdrawn or reduced until the person's care needs have been assessed (or reassessed) against revised eligibility criteria. Any reduction in, withdrawal of, or refusal to provide services must not leave individuals at severe physical risk.**

How to contact social services

If the family doctor has not referred your relative's case to social services, you can contact the department directly to request an assessment.

In most parts of England and Wales, the social services department is listed in the phone book under the name of the local authority. In some parts of the country, local authorities have reorganised into new unitary authorities, particularly in former county council areas. In Scotland, the department will be under 'social work' under the name of the local authority. In Northern Ireland, you need to contact your local Health and Social Services Board.

If you have problems, your local Age Concern organisation will be able to point you in the right direction.

If your relative is in hospital, contact the social work department at the hospital and tell them that you would like your relative to be assessed so that help can be arranged for when she is discharged.

Persuading your relative to use services

The success of the care plan depends on the expertise of those introducing it and on the tact and sensitivity of the workers. Sometimes you may find that your relative is reluctant to accept the help that is offered – what do you do then?

▪ Try to involve other people in talking to your relative – the community psychiatric nurse, social worker or GP. She may feel happier talking through the situation with someone other than her carer, who is knowledgeable about dementia and about the services being offered.

▪ Can you identify why your relative is saying no? Is there a real fear behind it, or does it stem from a denial of her failing abilities?

▪ Sometimes another person can help your relative to see that *you* need a break.

▪ A person with dementia can become suspicious or misinterpret events. A new person or new environment needs to be introduced gradually, with repeated explanations.

If you can't get the help you need

Joan

'My mother is 92, blind, incontinent at times, barely mobile and sometimes thinks I am her mother. I find you are strictly alone at every crisis. It is one long battle after another. Mum has already had a wait of nine months for a wheelchair.'

You may be lucky and live in an area where community care services are well coordinated and provide you with the help you want. But in some areas services that should be available are not getting to the people who need them most.

If you are unhappy with the way you and your relative are treated, and you are not able to resolve the difficulties in another way, you may wish to make a complaint. You might do this if, for example:

■ There is a long delay before your relative can be assessed.
■ You do not feel that the help offered is enough to meet your relative's needs.
■ You do not feel that the help offered is enough to meet your needs as the carer.

You can invoke the official complaints procedure by writing to the social services department setting out the details of your complaint. Local authorities are required to have a complaints procedure. This must have three stages:

The informal stage Staff and managers of the service try to resolve the matter through informal discussion with the complainant (the person making the complaint). If this fails, the complainant registers a formal complaint in writing. The social services department should offer information about how to do this and who to write to, and if necessary offer assistance.

The report or formal stage The department should carry out an investigation within 28 days, or explain why this time scale is not possible. In any case, a reply must be given within three months. If the complainant is still not satisfied, the complaint goes before a review panel.

The review or panel stage At least one member of the panel must be independent of the local authority. The complainant may be accompanied by a non-lawyer representative; if necessary, the department should help the complainant by supplying an advocate – someone to speak on their behalf. The panel hears the complaint and the evidence and a recommendation is passed to the Director of Social Services.

If you are not satisfied with the outcome of the complaint, the matter can be referred to the Local Government Ombudsman (address on p 112), who looks into cases of maladministration in local government.

For more *i*nformation

ⓘ Carers National Association Factsheet *A fair deal for carers: your guide to getting services.*

ⓘ *The Community Care Handbook* (2nd edition), published by Age Concern Books (details on p 117).

ⓘ The Carers National Association has a **CarersLine** – 0171-490 8898.

ⓘ Age Concern England Factsheet 41 *Local authority assessments for community care services.*

Getting a break from caring

If you are the main carer for someone with dementia, the best way to avoid a crisis is to ensure that you have time to yourself to recover your energies and to pursue your own life away from the person who is ill. Without a break, your own reserves will wear down very quickly and you may become ill or exhausted. There are various options for what is known as 'respite care'. You may find you use them all during the course of the illness.

Greta

'I was under a lot of mental strain and needed help. The social worker came to visit us at home and handled the situation so well that my husband agreed to have a "carer" sit with him so that I could have time off to do some shopping. Later he agreed to day care one day a week, which enabled me to have a complete day of freedom. A nearby residential home has a good day centre attached to it. So gradually my husband has become used to the day centre, and having stayed in the home itself while I had a holiday he has now agreed to stay there one week each month. I am so grateful. I leave him with complete peace of mind.'

Different types of respite care

Your social worker, GP or community psychiatric nurse will be able to tell you about the options for respite care in your area. Services vary hugely between different areas of the country but the following should be on offer:

Help at home Someone comes to your relative's home to look after her while you take a break. This can be for a few hours or for longer periods of time. The people who offer this service may be called 'sitters' or 'care attendants'.

Day breaks away from home The person with dementia attends a day centre, which may be attached to a residential home or nursing home, or a day hospital. Transport is usually arranged and you may be able to get some help in getting your relative ready to leave in the morning.

Longer breaks away from home The person with dementia has regular stays of two to six weeks in a local care home or hospital. This is sometimes known as 'phased care'. See pages 70–73 on the different types of care home and pages 74–77 on looking for a good home.

As the illness progresses you will probably need regular help on a daily basis, for example someone coming in to help you get your relative dressed and bathed, someone to stay with your relative when you go out shopping, and a proper break every six weeks or so. Obviously what you and your relative need will depend on your situation and the severity of her condition, but most carers say that a regular break is essential in order to keep going.

Paying for respite care

If your relative goes into a care home for respite care, the local authority may carry out a means test (taking into account only her own resources) to decide how much she should contribute towards the fees. (For the position for a couple when the spouse going into the care home has a private pension, see pp 73–74.)

However, if her stay is less than eight weeks, they may simply charge what appears 'reasonable' for her to pay. If you do not feel the charge is 'reasonable' you can ask the local authority to reduce or waive the charge. You can also make a complaint through the social services department's complaints procedure. If the respite care is provided by the NHS, it will be free.

Care inside or outside your own home?

Whether to arrange care inside or outside your home can be a hard decision. When you are looking for a service that suits your needs and those of the person you care for, you may have a difficult balancing act. On the one hand, many people with dementia become more confused when they are taken out of their own environment, and some may not be willing to attend a day centre. On the other hand, you may feel that you need time alone in your own home to relax and recuperate.

If you think it is best for your relative to be cared for in her own home, there are some agencies, most of them private, who will send someone either for a few hours or to live in while you go away. Ask your social worker or local Age Concern organisation if they know of any reputable agencies offering this service.

Having someone living in is generally a more expensive option than your relative going into a residential or nursing home. If your relative has been assessed by social services, and they are arranging services for her, this option may not be open to her because some local authorities place 'ceilings' or upper limits on the cost of care at home.

There are some pioneering schemes which help people to make the gradual transition from respite care in the person's own home to longer-term care outside the home. Some EMI registered residential homes (see p 71) offer day care, longer periods of respite care (a few weeks) and evening care. Gradually the person with dementia becomes used to the different environment, and if the time comes when she has to move into permanent care, the wrench is less heartrending.

If you are not fortunate enough to have such a scheme near you, you need to plan various ways of lightening the load and of getting away from the situation completely. This should form part of your social services assessment (see pp 48–51).

Making independent arrangements

If you do not want to involve social services, you can of course make your own arrangements with private agencies if you can afford to do so.

You can also contact voluntary organisations that run services such as day centres, lunch clubs, sitting schemes, support groups, help with transport or equipment loans. Others may provide advice and information. 'Voluntary' does not necessarily mean that the organisation is run by volunteers: it means it is independent of health and social services and is not run to make a profit.

One of the most extensive voluntary organisations that helps carers in a practical way is Crossroads Care, which can arrange for a care attendant to come to your home to look after your relative. To find out if there is a branch near you, contact the national address on page 111.

For more *i*nformation

 Age Concern England Factsheet 6 *Finding help at home.*

 Age Concern England Factsheet 41 *Local authority assessments for community care services.*

 Ask your **GP, health visitor**, **community psychiatric nurse** or ask other carers.

 Contact your **Council for Voluntary Service, Citizens Advice Bureau** or **Community Health Council/Health Council** (all listed in the phone book).

 Ask at the local **reference library**.

 If you attend a **place of worship**, ask for information about local groups.

4 The later stages of dementia

Caring for someone in the later stages of dementia presents new problems. The ill person may develop changes in personality and behaviour or he may become physically frail and need more intensive nursing. As one carer said, 'It was not so much a case of crisis – it was more a case of straws to break the camel's back.' It is this gradual wearing down of reserves that is so tiring: you learn to manage one situation and then the next difficulty comes along.

This chapter looks at some of the problems of caring for someone with advanced dementia. It discusses three areas that often mark a crisis point for carers – lack of mobility, aggression and incontinence – and looks at how to keep an eye on your relative's general health. The second part looks at the options for residential or nursing home care when it is no longer possible to care at home.

Karen

'Their weekly visits are very tiring for my husband and myself, so we have sympathy for my brother caring for her full time.'

'My brother cares for his wife, Sue, who has Alzheimer's. We have noticed on their regular weekly visits how Sue's condition has deteriorated notice-ably during the last two years, and wonder how much longer my brother can cope. Sue doesn't know our Christian names and sometimes doesn't know who her husband is, or her only daughter – although strange to say she recognises one of our children, who was her favourite as a little boy. At times she can be very truculent and the GP has to be called to calm her down.

'Their weekly visits are very tiring for my husband and myself, so we have sympathy for my brother caring for her full time. After eight hours in her company yesterday we were mentally and physically exhausted. She didn't sit down at all, but paraded from room to room. I noticed her hands were very sore and gave her a jar of hand cream. I explained 'Put some on your hands', but she promptly put it all over her face. I repeated the process and again all over the face it went. In the end I had to rub her hands, then she rounded on me, 'I know how to do it.' She powdered her nose in the lounge and put on lipstick and couldn't find the bathroom (across the hall) four times each in the space of an hour. She opened her handbag and purse no less than 20 times.

'She will butter bread and wash up whilst here but will do nothing at home. Telling the time is no problem but she cannot relate it to the time of day. At night she wanders downstairs to the toilet – there's one upstairs but she can't find it. She has lived in the same house for about 40 years.

'Recently I took her to buy a new dress. We chose several for her to try and she started getting undressed before we reached the changing room. In a cafe or public toilets, I always have to be in attendance: she has left taps running, doesn't close toilet doors … In short, she has to be monitored 24 hours a day.'

Problems in the later stages of dementia

Looking after someone in the later stages of dementia presents the carer with new difficulties. You may by now have become accustomed to the demands of a person who cannot hold an ordinary conversation and sometimes forgets who you are. But the personality changes and physical deterioration that often accompany the later stages of the illness can introduce a different level of stress for the carer and wider family.

Loss of mobility

No two people with dementia are alike: some become very active in the later stages of the illness, others appear to be very passive and unwilling to move. It is important to keep your relative active as long as possible, but as soon as he does become unable to walk or to move easily, do ask your occupational therapist for advice about adaptations to the home.

With more restricted mobility, many people lose weight; some research suggests that the disease itself may contribute to muscle wasting.

Falls

Stiffness and poor balance can make a person with dementia more prone to falls. You will already have taken the precautions outlined on pages 23–24 to make the home as safe as possible. If your relative now needs your assistance to walk or get out of bed, you will need to be very careful with your own back. Ask the district nurse or a physiotherapist to demonstrate ways of helping your relative without causing undue strain on you. If your relative does have a fall:

- Stay calm.
- Check for any injury or immediate pain.
- Continue to watch for any swelling, bruises or signs of distress and call the doctor if you are worried.

Pressure sores

People who are unable to leave their bed may develop pressure sores. If you notice red patches on your relative's skin which do not disappear after a few hours, you should contact the district nurse immediately. Treated early, they will not be a problem; left untreated, they can become badly infected and your relative may need to be admitted to hospital.

Here are some measures you can take to avoid pressure sores:

- Ensure your relative exercises regularly and encourage him to move around when sitting or lying.
- If your relative is incontinent, try to ensure that he does not

stay in wet clothes or a wet bed (see below for more advice about incontinence).

- Avoid tight clothing or bedding which can hamper circulation.
- Keep your relative cool and in loose-fitting clothes so that heat and sweat do not build up.
- Always dry him well after a bath or a wash, using a patting action rather than rubbing, which could damage the skin.
- Ensure your relative has a well-balanced diet that will keep the skin as healthy as possible.

For more *i*nformation

i Alzheimer's Disease Society Advice Sheet 13 *Pressure sores*.

Loss of bladder or bowel control

Incontinence is not inevitable: it does not happen to everyone with dementia. If your relative becomes incontinent, consult your doctor immediately: many cases of incontinence are treatable. Even if the condition cannot be treated, there is much that can be done to help you manage your workload and to make the whole situation less difficult for you both.

If a person with dementia does become incontinent, it can often feel like the last shreds of their independence and dignity are being stripped away. You may feel strongly about cleaning up after someone and it is important to acknowledge these feelings.

Rita

'Yesterday my ultimate fear happened. Double incontinence. I knew it would come at some point, but I thought, "Oh, that's years away yet." When I realised what a mess she was in, my reaction was – selfish as it must seem – to burst into tears. It was the initial shock that my mother! my mother! had actually messed herself. I decided that I needed help and called on Mum's sister. She calmly got Mum in the shower and changed her.'

What causes incontinence?

There are many causes of urinary incontinence which may be treatable, for example:

■ a urinary tract infection;
■ prostate gland trouble in men;
■ diuretics used for heart conditions or drugs which make the person more confused;
■ weakening muscles;
■ severe constipation, which puts pressure on the urinary system. For tips about how to tell when someone is constipated, see page 68.

Incontinence of the bowels can similarly be caused by treatable conditions such as constipation or an infection.

Who can help?

Once the GP has addressed any medical cause, he or she may pass you on to the district or community nurse, health visitor or continence adviser for further help. If you wish, you can contact the continence adviser directly. Continence advisers are specialist nurses who work with people who have incontinence problems. They will look at what is causing the problem and help you to find a solution or refer you to someone else for further help. If you have difficulty in finding out about a continence adviser, you can get in touch with the Continence Foundation; they also offer general information and advice. Or you can ring the Incontinence Information Helpline (details on p 112).

Equipment and supplies

Ask social services whether the local authority runs an incontinence laundry service, and check with the district nurse if the health authority provides any help with this. Find out what your local health authority might provide in the way of incontinence pads or other supplies.

If you are considering buying equipment, you might find it useful to contact your local Disabled Living Centre if there is one (listed in the telephone directory). They will often have samples of equipment and clothing and can give you advice on where to buy them.

If you prefer to borrow equipment, your social services department may be able to help. Some local organisations have information on loans of commodes and some other equipment: the Red Cross, Women's Royal Voluntary Service (WRVS), St John Ambulance and Age Concern.

Managing incontinence

People with dementia may behave strangely when they are incontinent. They may, for example, urinate in odd places like a drawer or a plant pot, or they may blame someone else for leaving wet clothes on their chair. Upsetting as this is for you, try not to get angry. Instead, talk it over with the district nurse or continence adviser. There may be a number of steps you can take to help you to deal with the problem:

■ Take your relative to the toilet at regular intervals. Make a diary of his routine so that you can make sure you take him to the toilet at a time he would naturally want to go.

■ Look out for signs, such as restless movements, getting up and down, or pulling at clothes.

■ Make sure he wears clothes that are easy to unfasten and to take off.

■ If your relative cannot get to the bathroom in time you could ask the district nurse or social services for a commode, or buy or borrow one.

■ If your relative has difficulty finding the bathroom – especially in a new setting – put a large sign on the door.

■ If your relative cannot communicate easily, you (or a sitter) may miss what he is asking for. Learn to understand what he is trying to say.

■ Cut down fluids in the evening, but make sure he drinks well the rest of the day.

■ Use a bedside commode. Night lights in the bathroom and bedroom can also be a help.

■ If regular toileting does not work, you may need to use incontinence pads and pants – ask the district nurse or continence adviser for advice.

For more *i*nformation

i Age Concern England Factsheet 23 *Help with incontinence.*

i Alzheimer's Disease Society Advice Sheet 3 *Incontinence.*

i **The Continence Foundation** (address on p 110) offers general information and advice.

Dealing with aggression

Gwen

'It started about seven years ago, he would say he didn't know what I was talking about (but everyone else did!). I looked upon this as rudeness. He had been mildly aggressive for some time, which I just thought was a hot temper, inherited from his mother. Once he ran the Hoover into my feet. Another time, waiting to be called up for a flight at the airport, he punched me, in public, for no particular reason, and waiting for the airport bus, he whacked my legs with his stick. I still just took these incidents to be frustration. After the holiday, the aggression became worse and we went to the doctor. It was then I realised his brain was affected.'

It can be very shocking and upsetting when the person you care for becomes angry and aggressive, especially when this behaviour is out of character. This behaviour may start quite early on in the illness or it may suddenly develop later. Others, of course, never show any signs of anger and may express their frustrations in quite different ways.

Often the anger is directed at the person closest – but that does not mean that your relative is angry *with* you or that he hates you. Remember that his brain is damaged, and anger cannot be interpreted in the usual way.

Your relative may be getting angry because of:

Misunderstanding He may not know what is going on, or misinterpret what is happening. If he is aware of his declining abilities, he may, for example, accuse others of stealing his possessions, rather than face the difficult truth that his memory is failing him.

What you can do Take time to explain what is happening in simple sentences. Use a calm tone and a reassuring manner.

Feeling pressured Everyday demands become progressively more difficult to manage and simple tasks may become impossible. An outburst may result if you try to hurry your relative, saying 'Put your coat on now', or if you try to stop him doing something with 'Don't do that'.

What you can do Slow down your routine so that you do not have to hurry. Avoid direct requests if they cause distress and try to find ways to get things done by using persuasion and distraction.

Feeling frustrated Situations where the person with dementia feels trapped or humiliated – perhaps with having to accept help with simple tasks such as dressing and going to the toilet – can also trigger aggression.

What you can do Even if it takes a long time, try to find ways for your relative to carry on doing things independently. Be positive and praise achievements.

Unfamiliar people or surroundings A change in routine, or unknown faces or noises, may make your relative fearful and upset.

What you can do Explain to others that he may not know who they are and that sudden movements or noises may be frightening.

These tactics may not work. It is not your fault if they don't. When your relative gets angry, try not to be drawn into an argument – you may have to leave the room to take a deep breath and calm yourself down. If you do respond, it is only human, so don't give yourself a hard time, but do try and talk it over with someone who you know will be sympathetic.

To be hit, verbally abused or threatened by someone you are caring for hurts deeply, so don't expect yourself to manage alone. Sometimes a friend or a professional helper can encourage the person with dementia to behave in a different way.

Jess

'Very unexpectedly, for no apparent reason, rages occurred, some of which were very frightening. The rages exhausted him, and he would go into a profound sleep, waking up hours later amenable again.'

Jim

'She went through various stages of aggression over the years – the worst one being about four to five years ago when I did not dare turn my back on her. At this stage I hid all the carving knives for a period of time. As it was, I was pushed down the stairs one day.'

Here are some tips for handling an outburst as calmly as possible:

Don't argue or take personal offence.

Do stay calm and try not to show fear.

Do try to defuse the situation by suggesting doing something else – forgetfulness is an advantage and your relative may move on and forget his anger.

Don't try to restrain your relative unless absolutely necessary – give him space to calm down.

Don't use punishments – your relative cannot learn by experience.

What about you?

Paula

'His illness changed his personality, making him cross and antisocial, but it was his aggressiveness that was the problem. I began to be frightened of him. Especially at night, he would start to lash out – not like my Bill. Just as I dozed off to sleep, he would start again. You keep it to yourself, but in the end I told the doctor as Bill wasn't a man like that, it was alien to his nature. At that time, I had a feeling of hate for this man. We seemed to be forever arguing, which wasn't like us. I had tried everything to please and couldn't win.'

Sue

'He has terrible nightmares and I have to sleep in the same bed so that I can get hold of his pyjamas before he throws himself out of bed. Sometimes he gets out of bed and tries to run, so I have to hold him the best way I can, but he becomes violent and has hurt me many times. Occasionally I have to phone for my son when I cannot manage him alone, as it takes the two of us a couple of hours to get him to bed.'

If aggressive episodes are frequent, and if you are in any physical danger yourself, it is essential for you to talk to a professional. Your GP, community psychiatric nurse or psychogeriatrician may be able to suggest ways to handle the problem. It is generally best not to treat the aggression with drugs, but in some cases it becomes the only option. It is then important that the treatment is kept under regular review as the drugs could add to your relative's confusion. In some cases, the situation is so serious that you may have to start thinking about alternative forms of care.

Dealing with routine health problems

In the later stages of dementia, when your relative cannot tell you that something is wrong, it becomes particularly important to keep an eye on his general health. If he lives on his own, he may not eat and drink properly.

Dental treatment

Your relative should continue to receive regular dental check-ups. Even people who are moderately forgetful can neglect their teeth or their dentures and develop oral infections, and those may not be obvious to you just from looking in your relative's mouth.

Try to find an understanding dentist who will work slowly and gently with your relative. If necessary, ask for your relative to be referred to the Community Dental Service, who are trained to work with people whose understanding of what is happening to them is limited.

Problems with vision

You should ensure that your relative has regular eye examinations. Ask the Health Authority (Health Board in Scotland) whether there are any local opticians who are experienced in working with people who have dementia. If you suspect that he has a problem with his eyes, arrange for him to be seen by an opthalmologist.

A person whose brain is impaired can also have difficulties with distinguishing between similar colour intensities. Thus a dark handrail on a white wall will be easier to use than a white one. Prints and patterns can also be confusing.

Problems with hearing

As with a vision problem, it can be hard to distinguish between problems of thinking and problems of hearing. If you suspect a hearing problem, ask your GP to refer your relative to an audiologist at an Ear, Nose and Throat (ENT) clinic.

Constipation

If your relative appears to be in pain, has a problem with wind or headaches and there is no fever or cough, constipation may be the problem. A person with dementia may not be able to remember when he last moved his bowels and may not connect the pain with constipation. If your relative is living alone, he may be eating low-fibre foods that slow down bowel activity. If you suspect constipation is a problem, consult the GP, who will confirm whether or not your relative needs treatment.

Residential or nursing home care

Doreen

'When the specialist saw him for assessment, she said I was at breaking point and had done well to cope as long as I had. By this time, my son and my husband's family were saying, "You can't go on with him like this."'

When you have done all you can

You may have reached the point where the person you care for needs more help or support than you can provide. This may be after your relative has had a fall or has been admitted to hospital for some reason. Perhaps your own health is failing. The time has come to think about a care home. This is a major decision and a difficult one.

If the situation has not already reached a crisis point and you have time to consider the options, you may want to consider whether any of these might help before you make the decision to move your relative to a home.

A regular break Sometimes a break from caring on a regular basis can help you regain your health and enable you to think about the future. For information on respite care, see pages 54–57. Respite care can also be a way of introducing your relative to day care in a different environment, with a view to eventually moving into a care home permanently. Speak to your doctor, social worker or local Alzheimer's Disease Society about how to find respite care.

A medical assessment If your relative has not already had a proper medical assessment, contact the GP and request one. Changes in your relative's behaviour or in his health which are causing you problems may be caused by drugs or by a treatable medical condition.

69

A social services assessment If you have not contacted social services before, ask them to make an assessment of your relative's needs (see pp 48–51). The person making the assessment can also advise you on the options for residential care if this is what you feel is needed.

Advice from a voluntary organisation Sometimes health and social services professionals have strong views of their own and you want to talk to someone else who can give you a different perspective. Your local Age Concern, Alzheimer's Disease Society or carers' group should be able to help you talk through the options and guide you in the right direction for further help.

Arranging admission to a care home

The most usual route into a residential or nursing home is directly from hospital. A person with dementia is admitted after a crisis in their health and it becomes evident that the carer is not able to continue caring for the person at home. In this instance, the hospital social work team makes an assessment and will probably suggest a few homes to the carer to go and visit.

If the person with dementia is not in hospital, social services are still likely to be involved. If the local authority is being asked to help with the fees, the entry into a home will be via the social services assessment and social services will help find a home and arrange the place. If your relative has sufficient funds to pay for himself, you can find a home independently – but social services can still offer you information and advice.

But if you are worried that your relative may need financial help from the State in the future, you should ask social services to assess his needs and make the arrangements with the home. Even if he has enough funds to pay for many years, and never needs State funding, you may find the assessment process helpful in identifying suitable homes.

Which kind of care home?

There are two kinds of care home: residential homes and nursing homes.

Residential homes

Residential homes may also be referred to as rest homes, old people's homes or Part III homes (Part IV homes in Scotland). They are for people who need help with personal care and day-to-day activities rather than nursing care.

Residential homes run by local authority social services departments are often called Part III homes; private individuals or companies and voluntary organisations also run homes. All homes must be inspected by the social services Inspection and Registration Unit at least twice a year. Homes run by private or voluntary organisations are also registered by this unit. Small residential homes (for fewer than four people) must also register under a simplified process. They may also be inspected, but this is not a regular requirement. Copies of inspection reports should be made available on request, but you should also consider visiting the homes yourself.

For people with dementia, the home may be called an EMI (Elderly Mentally Infirm) registered home. The term EMI is currently being changed in some areas to 'mentally disordered older people'. These homes will often provide similar care to that in a nursing home, but they may be cheaper.

Finding out about local residential homes

If you have a query about a residential home, or need information about what homes there are in your area, you should contact the Inspection and Registration Unit of the social services department of your local council, whose phone number will be listed in the local telephone directory. Once your relative has been assessed by the social services department, they should suggest homes which would meet her needs.

Many residential and nursing homes won't accept people with Alzheimer's disease. The Alzheimer's Disease Society (address on p 109) has a national database of care homes, which it can search for those that take people with dementia.

Nursing homes

Nursing homes are for people who need full-time nursing care. Most nursing homes are run privately or by voluntary organisations. All nursing homes have to be registered with the Health Authority (Health Board in Scotland) and inspected at least twice a year. The person in charge of the home must be either a registered medical practitioner or a qualified nurse. It is planned that Health Authorities will have to make public their inspection reports on the homes they visit – check with the Health Authority to find out if their inspection reports are available.

Finding out about local nursing homes

Your first call should be to the Registration and Inspection Unit for Nursing Homes. This will probably be listed in your local telephone directory under your health authority. If you can't find it, contact your Community Health Council (called a Health Council in Scotland), also listed in the local directory. All private nursing homes must be registered with the local health authority – *never* use one that is not registered.

Once the social services department has assessed your relative as needing a place in a nursing home, they should also suggest suitable homes.

The Registration and Inspection Officer for Nursing Homes will be able to give you information about which private nursing homes are registered in your area. Although the officer cannot recommend individual homes, he or she can advise you about which homes cater for people with dementia. Some health authorities have produced their own standards of care in addition to national guidelines. Ask if you can have a copy of these – they may be useful when you visit individual homes.

Other organisations that can help you find a nursing home are the Alzheimer's Disease Society, the Elderly Accommodation Counsel, Counsel and Care and the Relatives Association (addresses on pp 109–113).

Note Some private placement agencies work on a commission basis,
so their advice may not be impartial. They may also charge for information which is freely available from other agencies.

Dual-registered homes

Some homes are 'dual-registered', which means that they combine
the services offered by residential and nursing homes. This may be
an advantage if your relative's care needs are likely to increase, to
include nursing care, as this may mean she does not have to move
from one home to another. You may need to check how the home
defines 'nursing care' as this may mean paying a higher fee.

Paying for residential and nursing home care

Residential and nursing homes can be very expensive. High charges
do not necessarily reflect better quality care, but they may mean
more luxurious surroundings.

If your relative has capital assets of £16,000 or less, he may get
help with the cost from social services. He will have to have his
needs assessed. If, as a result, social services decide to arrange a
place in a care home, they will be responsible for meeting the full
cost but they will assess your relative's income and savings to see
how much he should pay towards the cost. This is called a **means
test** or **financial assessment**. Your relative may also qualify for
some support from the Department of Social Security – the people carrying out the assessment should advise you – but this will
be counted as part of his income for purposes of the financial
assessment.

If you have enough funds to make your own arrangements, you
can of course negotiate directly with the care homes of your
choice. It may nevertheless be wise to ask social services to assess
your relative's needs, as explained on page 75.

For many people, the financial implications of going into a care
home come as a shock. This can be particularly so if the person
going into a care home is one of a couple and has the majority of
the couple's income. However, the rules were changed in 1996 and

again in 1997 so that the local authority ignore half of any private pension when they are calculating the resident's contribution to the fees. They will do this if at least half of the private pension is being handed over to the spouse. The spouse must not be living in the same care home as the resident. It does not apply to unmarried couples. By 'private pension' we mean a personal or occupational pension or a payment from a retirement annuity. See Age Concern's Factsheet 39 *Paying for care in a residential or nursing home if you have a partner*.

For more *i*nformation

i Alzheimer's Disease Society Information Sheet 21 *Residential and nursing home care.*

i Alzheimer Scotland – Action on Dementia *A positive choice – choosing long-stay care for a person with dementia* (for readers in Scotland).

i Age Concern England Factsheet 10 *Local authority charging procedures for residential and nursing home care.*

i Age Concern England Factsheet 29 *Finding residential or nursing home accommodation.*

i Age Concern England Factsheet 39 *Paying for care in a residential or nursing home if you have a partner.*

i For information about long-term care insurance policies, see 'Take a long-term view', in February 1997 *Which?* (available from the Consumers' Association, 2 Marylebone Road, London NW1 4DF. Tel: 0171-830 6000).

i For more help and advice, contact your local **Citizens Advice Bureau** or **Age Concern** organisation – as well as the social services department.

Looking for a good home

If the situation has reached a crisis point, you may feel under pressure to make a decision in a hurry, but try to resist doing so. It may be a hard time to be practical, but there are many questions to consider because you are looking for a complete care service for your relative, not just reasonable accommodation.

In some parts of the country, it can be hard to find a suitable care home, but don't be tempted to accept the first one with a vacancy. If your relative has been assessed by social services as being in need of residential or nursing home care, it is their responsibility to find a suitable home. So, even if your relative has enough money to pay the home's fees, it may still be worth asking social services for a community care assessment.

You and your relative should expect the same rights and choices as when you are living in your own home. Residents are entitled to a service that offers privacy, dignity, autonomy, choice and fulfilment.

In meeting these standards, a good quality home should provide:

- a full written contract;
- a pre-agreed care plan;
- information about how the home operates;
- a complaints procedure.

These are not legal requirements, but a home offering these is showing a willingness to deliver a service that respects the rights and wishes of the people who use it.

When you visit a home

It is often helpful to visit a home with a trusted friend or family member. You may be shocked by the other residents: everyone else tends to look more ill than your own relative. This is probably not the case, but it is often the first impression.

Some questions are essential to ask when you visit a home if you have not already asked them, for example:

- Is the home registered?
- Is there a contract and a written care plan?
- Does the home belong to any professional trade association?

Other questions will be dictated by your and your relative's priorities, since everybody's needs are different. So first of all ask yourself, or discuss with other members of the family: What kind of home do I want for my relative? Here is a sample of questions you might want to ask:

- How many staff are on duty and what is the ratio of staff to residents?
- What kind of training do the staff have?
- Are residents encouraged to do as much as they can themselves and to maintain choice in their day-to-day lives?
- Can residents bring their own possessions into the home?
- How is the laundry service organised?
- Do residents eat when and what they choose? Can they prepare snacks and drinks for themselves?
- Can visitors come at any time? Can they stay for a meal or overnight?
- What activities are on offer?
- How much of the home is communal? Are there separate rooms for television and for quiet activities?
- Are there any outings arranged into the local community?
- Can your relative stay until he dies?

You could also ask how residents and their relatives are kept informed about changes and day-to-day developments in the home. Does the home appear to encourage open communication and involvement or are people expected to 'fit in'? Does the home set out rigorous standards in a Charter of Rights?

Draw up your own checklist of questions before you visit and don't feel embarrassed about asking lots of questions – most homes would expect you to do so. If you can, talk to residents and staff in private. You could also ask to talk to relatives of residents.

For more *i*nformation

 More comprehensive checklists are available free of charge in the following publications:

 How to Choose a Good Care Home, published by British Federation of Care Home Proprietors.

i Counsel and Care Factsheet 5 *What to look for in a private or voluntary registered home*.

i Age Concern England Factsheet 29 *Finding residential and nursing home accommodation*.

What to look for when you visit

As well as asking questions, the point of making a personal visit is to see for yourself how a home operates. Here are some things to look out for as you go round:

- Do staff treat the residents with respect and dignity?
- How do they address residents?
- Are the buildings and grounds well maintained and cared for?
- Does the home look and smell clean?
- Is physical access good?
- Is there an easily accessible garden or outdoor area?
- Are toilets and bathrooms equipped with aids and designed for privacy?
- Do residents look well cared for?
- Does the home have adequate stair lifts and fire escapes?

A trial stay

Even if you are completely satisfied with the home you should try to arrange a trial stay for at least a month to allow your relative to get to know the home and the home to get to know your relative. Do not sell any property or give up rented accommodation until you are sure the move is definite.

Your feelings when the decision is made

Your relative moving into a home may mark the beginning of a period of bereavement for you as the carer. Guilt, sadness and anger may be mixed with a feeling of relief. You may find it hard to sleep and the days may suddenly seem empty and long. Some people feel that allowing the person they care for to go into a home is a mark of failure, and you may feel you have let your relative down even though you know you have done all you can and the decision is for the best.

Pam

'My profound physical exhaustion has eased, and in its place I have feelings of desolation and inadequacy and an ever-present financial worry which, after our efforts to provide for an independent old age, I did not expect. Not least, there is also the daily trauma of leaving him.'

When the transition is more gradual it gives you, and the person you care for, time to adjust to the change.

Naina

'Before my mother went to the home, she went about three times a week in a minibus to get used to the place. The home care assistant helped me get her ready. She didn't want to go, which upset me, but I was told she was okay when she got there.'

For some carers, this final stage can be a great relief and a very positive experience – one which feels right for everybody concerned.

Joan

'She was in the old folks' home for just three months. They were so kind and it was near to where I live, so I was able to see her every day and was with her when she passed away so peacefully.'

For more *i*nformation

- *ⓘ* *Finding and paying for residential and nursing home care*, published by Age Concern Books (details on p 115).

- *ⓘ* *Residential Care? The options for later life*, published by The Stationery Office. Available from Age Concern Scotland (address on p 114).

5 Making legal and financial decisions

As the person you are caring for becomes more confused, so her power to make important legal and financial decisions diminishes and it is usually necessary for the carer or other family member to assume these responsibilities on her behalf. The earlier you organise this, the better it is for all parties: if your relative is still in the early stages of dementia, she will be able to participate in discussions and arrangements. Later on, knowing that you are carrying out her wishes will give you peace of mind.

This chapter looks at how to take over management of your relative's financial affairs when this becomes necessary. It also looks at the costs of caring and the various kinds of financial help that may be available to you and your relative. Finally it discusses making a Will and drawing up a 'living will'.

Anne

'If carers encourage the people they care for to take out an enduring power of attorney soon enough, none of this stress need occur.'

'Our solicitor never mentioned anything about my husband taking out an enduring power of attorney whereby you appoint someone to see to your affairs if you are unable to. I can't stress enough how important this is. We spoke to my husband in hospital when they told us he had multi-infarct dementia and would not get better. I had for some time been doing his job of paying the bills, writing cheques and so on, but my son and I thought we should get power of attorney. The solicitor was willing to draw up the document but the hospital would not allow it. I know Eric understood then – he asked us to take care of everything, he didn't want to be worried with anything. "You do it," he said. They moved him from that hospital to another one for a further six weeks; by that time his health had really deteriorated. We were told we would have to apply to the Court of Protection instead of getting power of attorney. Nobody I knew had heard of it, and another worry was that they were wanting to put Eric in a nursing home costing £300 per week.

'My local carers' group had the address and phone number of the Court of Protection so I phoned. After much help it was felt that in my case, I would need to apply to the Court of Protection only if I wanted to sell the bungalow as I would need my husband's signature.

'But if carers encourage the people they care for to take out an enduring power of attorney soon enough, none of this stress need occur. I gather that applying to the Court of Protection can be time-consuming and costly.'

Managing someone else's finances

As dementia progresses, the ill person will need someone else to take over her affairs and to make arrangements on her behalf. This can happen informally, but there are ways in which the law can be helpful in putting this on a more formal footing. This is important where money and property are concerned.

Acting as an agent

An 'agent' is someone who collects pensions or benefits on behalf of another person. This can be useful in the early stages of dementia, where the ill person is still able to look after her own money with some help. If this is a long-term arrangement, you can obtain an identification card from your local benefits Agency or complete form API *A Helping Hand: How you can help somebody with a disability claim the social security benefits due to them* (AP1 (W) for people living in Wales).

Acting as an appointee

Once the person with dementia reaches the point where she is no longer able to act for herself, another person may be 'appointed' to claim pension and benefits on her behalf and to spend them on her needs.

If you want to be an 'appointee', you should contact your local Benefits Agency. You should be visited by an officer who will want to be assured that:

- Your relative is indeed unable to manage her own affairs.
- You are the right person to take over and will use the money for her well-being.
- You fully understand your responsibilities.

Power of attorney

An **ordinary power of attorney** is a legal document by which you appoint someone to act on your behalf to manage your financial affairs. It is no longer valid when the person becomes mentally incapable of understanding what is going on (except in Scotland, see p 84). So your relative will need to take out an **enduring power of attorney** if you are to be able to manage her affairs once she has become mentally incapable.

Drawing up an enduring power of attorney (EPA) is a legal option open to anyone over the age of 18 in England and Wales (Scottish readers, please see p 84) who is mentally capable and wants to plan ahead in the event of becoming mentally incapacitated. The person (donor) grants powers to another person or persons (the attorney or attorneys) to deal with the donor's financial affairs. The attorney can then do anything the donor can do (within the provisions of the EPA Act 1985), such as signing cheques, or buying or selling property.

Even after a diagnosis such as Alzheimer's disease, it is still possible to grant an EPA provided the donor fully understands what is happening. If in doubt, seek advice from a doctor and a solicitor.

How do you go about it?

- ▨ You should consult a solicitor about preparing an EPA or obtain a special form from a law stationers.
- ▨ Donor and attorney must sign the form in the presence of an independent witness – not necessarily at the same time or with the same witness.
- ▨ Once the attorney believes that the donor is or is becoming mentally incapable, the attorney must apply to the Protection Division of the Public Trust Office immediately to register the EPA. Notice of intention to register should be given to the donor and specified relatives, using forms obtainable from the Public Trust Office or law stationers; the Public Trustee deals with any objections and decides whether to register the EPA. Once the EPA is registered, the attorney can act or continue to act for the donor.

In certain circumstances it is possible to register an EPA without notifying the donor – you may feel that your relative would be upset at receiving a document stating that she is no longer capable of managing her own affairs. If you wish to do this, you should contact the Public Trust Office for advice.

For more help

ⓘ **LawNet** is a group of law firms recommended by the Alzheimer's Disease Society (address on p 109) to deal with legal and financial problems arising from dementia. Send an sae to the national office for the list.

The Court of Protection

If your relative has not made an enduring power of attorney and she is no longer capable of doing so, the only way for you to take over management of her financial affairs is to apply to the Court of Protection if you live in England or Wales or the Office of Care and Protection in Northern Ireland (Scottish readers, see p 84). The Court exists to look after the financial affairs and property of people who, because of 'mental disorder', cannot manage for themselves.

The Court can appoint a **receiver**, usually the nearest relative, to administer the person's affairs. If no close relative is willing to take on the responsibility, the receiver can be someone else, for example a representative of the local authority, solicitor or bank manager.

If the person's assets are less than £5,000 it may not be necessary to appoint a receiver. Instead, the Court may issue a **short order** or a **direction** that the person's assets should be used in a certain way.

To make an application to the Court of Protection, write to or telephone the Enquiries Branch, Public Trust Office (address on p 111). Your local Citizens Advice Bureau may also hold the forms. The person receiving your enquiry will want to know:

- your relationship to the person with dementia;
- the amount of financial assets to be controlled (especially if it is under £5,000).

If the person you care for lives in Northern Ireland, applications are made to the Office of Care and Protection (address on p 112) for appointment as a controller, whose role is the same as that of receiver.

For more *i*nformation

i Alzheimer's Disease Society Information Sheet 4 *Financial and legal arrangements.*

i Age Concern England Factsheet 22 *Legal arrangements for managing financial affairs.*

i *Enduring Power of Attorney* and *Handbook for Receivers*, both available free from the Court of Protection (address on p 111).

i *Managing Other People's Money*, published by Age Concern Books (details on p 118).

Managing someone else's money in Scotland

In Scotland a **power of attorney** granted after January 1991 can continue in force even after the donor has become mentally incapable of managing his or her own property and finances under the terms of the Law Reform (Miscellaneous Provisions) (Scotland) Act 1990. If the donor does not wish this to happen, this must be stated when power of attorney is granted. The services of a solicitor will be needed to prepare the power of attorney.

Negotiorum gestio This is a legal principle which assumes that when a person becomes incapable of managing their own affairs, someone else can act on their behalf because that person would have given authorisation if they were capable. However, the extent of this is not clear and not all organisations will accept this arrangement.

Curator bonis If your relative has not appointed a power of attorney and is mentally incapable of looking after her affairs or appointing someone else to look after them, then a curator bonis may have to be appointed. A curator bonis is an individual appointed by and responsible to the court. Usually a solicitor or accountant is appointed as curator (though not necessarily) and has to manage all the financial affairs and property of the person. The application to the court for a curator bonis to be appointed is prepared by a solicitor, usually on behalf of a close relative of the person. Having a curator appointed is expensive and any professional will charge an annual administration fee. It is therefore not recommended for people with less than £15,000 of capital.

In hospital The Health Board can take over responsibility for a person's finances if there is nobody else to do so. Alternatively, a carer or *curator bonis* can continue to manage the person's affairs. For sums in excess of £5,000 the hospital must obtain the consent of the Mental Welfare Commission for Scotland. A *curator bonis* is recommended for sums over £25,000. The hospital should use the money for the patient's benefit.

For more *i*nformation

ⓘ Contact **Alzheimer Scotland – Action on Dementia** (address on p 109), who also publish a guide called *Money and Legal Matters: A guide for carers*, which is free to carers.

ⓘ Age Concern Factsheet 22 *Legal Arrangements for Managing Financial Affairs* available from Age Concern Scotland (address on p 114).

ⓘ *Information for Families of Persons Subject to Curatory* leaflet available free from the Accountant of Court (address on page 109).

ⓘ *Dementia in the Community* free leaflet available from the Mental Welfare Commission for Scotland, K Floor, Argyle House, 3 Lady Lawson Street, Edinburgh EH3 9SH.

The costs of caring

Caring can have a serious impact on your finances. You may have had to give up work or take early retirement to look after your relative. You may be using your savings or those of your relative to buy in care or to pay for respite care. As you spend more time at home, gas and electricity bills increase, especially if your relative becomes incontinent and you are constantly washing sheets and clothes. Then there is the worry of meeting the costs of a care home if your relative's level of income and savings disqualifies her from local authority help.

If you are finding it hard to balance the books, you are not alone. A survey carried out by the Alzheimer's Disease Society in 1993 called *Deprivation and Dementia* showed that:

■ Of carers surveyed, 41 per cent were using their private savings and assets or had taken out a loan to meet the cost of caring for their relative.

■ Over a quarter paid more than £100 each month towards making up the shortfall in Government benefits for the care of their relative.

■ Nearly one in four carers anticipated having financial difficulties over the next two to three years.

■ Fourteen per cent were currently experiencing financial difficulties. Younger carers (aged 40–65) were most likely to be having financial problems.

■ Three per cent of carers had sold property to release capital.

Carers aged 80 or over are often particularly hard hit because they tend to have lower incomes than younger carers. The Alzheimer's Disease Society survey showed that for 20 per cent of the over-80s the costs of caring per week were more than the State Basic Pension for a single person – and that this expenditure was on top of normal daily living expenses.

Sources of financial help

If you are entitled to benefits, you should claim them. Attendance Allowance or the care component of Disability Living Allowance should be claimed by everyone who has dementia. All carers should check their entitlement to Invalid Care Allowance. Below are listed some of the main benefits and allowances. However, this is not an exhaustive list, so do ask for advice about your own situation.

Who to ask for advice

The Benefits Agency (which is part of the Department of Social Security) is responsible for paying benefits and is listed in your local telephone directory. You can phone your local office or ring the Benefits Agency freephone number for disabled people and their carers on 0800 88 22 00 (0800 22 06 74 for Northern Ireland).

You could also seek advice from other local organisations such as:

■ the Citizens Advice Bureau;
■ Age Concern;
■ the Alzheimer's Disease Society;
■ a carer's group;
■ a welfare rights unit.

Checklist of benefits you may be able to claim

Description
Attendance Allowance

For people who are physically or mentally ill and need help with personal care or who need supervision from someone else. Not means-tested; tax-free. If you become disabled under the age of 65, you should apply for Disability Living Allowance instead.

For more information
Age Concern England Factsheet 34 *Attendance Allowance and Disability Living Allowance*. Social security leaflet DS 702 and claim pack DS 2.

Description
Disability Living Allowance (DLA)

For people who become disabled and claim before the age of 65. A care component and a mobility component for people who cannot walk or who have difficulty getting about. Tax-free; not means-tested.

For more information
Age Concern England Factsheet 34 *Attendance Allowance and Disability Living Allowance*. Social security leaflet DS 704 and claim form DLA 1.

Description
Incapacity Benefit

Replaced Invalidity Benefit and Sickness Benefit in 1995. For people who are too sick or disabled to work. Based on National Insurance contributions. Normally stops at pension age.

For more information
Social security leaflet IB 202 (for new claimants).

Description
Severe Disablement Allowance

For severely disabled people who are unable to work but who have not paid enough NI contributions to get Incapacity Benefit. Claims can be made up to the age of 65.

For more information
Social security leaflet NI 252.

Description
Independent Living (1993) Fund

Can make payments to severely disabled people aged 16–65 who need to pay for care or household tasks in order to stay at home.

For more information
Contact your local social services department.

Description
Help with residential or nursing home fees

If you have savings of £16,000 or less, and the local authority has assessed you and agreed to arrange a place for you in a home, they will also means-test you to decide how much you need to pay towards the fees.

For more information
Age Concern England Factsheet 10 *Local authority charging procedures for residential and nursing home care.*

Description
Invalid Care Allowance (ICA)

For people who are unable to work full-time because they care for someone receiving a benefit such as Attendance Allowance for at least 35 hours a week. You will not qualify if you earn more than a certain amount. Some other benefits affected. Claims can be made up to the age of 65.

For more information
Social security claim pack DS 700.

Description
Jobseeker's Allowance

For people who have become unemployed and have paid NI contributions and are registered for Jobseeker's Allowance.

For more information
Social security leaflet JSA L5 or JSA L6 (for people near to or over age 60).

Description
Income Support

For people on a low income, with no more than £8,000 in savings (but the capital rules are different for people living in care homes), and not working more than 16 hours a week. A passport to other benefits and allowances.

For more information
Age Concern England Factsheet 25 *Income Support and the Social Fund.*
Social security leaflet IS 1.

Description
Carer premium

Not a benefit in its own right, but an extra sum paid to carers on Income
Support who qualify for Invalid Care Allowance.

For more information
As above.

Description
Housing Benefit (rent rebate in Northern Ireland)

Can provide help towards rent if you have a low income and savings of £16,000
or less.

For more information
Age Concern England Factsheet 17 *Housing Benefit and Council Tax
Benefit.* Social security leaflet RR 1.

Description
Council Tax Benefit (rate rebate in Northern Ireland)

Can provide help towards the Council Tax if you have a low income and savings of £16,000 or less.

For more information
Age Concern England Factsheet 17 *Housing Benefit and Council Tax
Benefit.* Contact the local authority.

Description
Council Tax discounts, exemptions and reductions

The Council Tax bill for disabled people or carers may also be affected by
these other schemes. Someone with dementia living alone may be exempt.

For more information
Age Concern England Factsheet 21 *The Council Tax and older people.*

Description
Social Fund

Can provide cash payments to cover extra exceptional expenses such as
funeral costs. For people on a low income with very limited savings.

For more information
Age Concern England Factsheet 25 *Income Support and the Social Fund.*
Social security leaflet SFL 2 *How the Social Fund can help you.*

Description
Help with house repairs

Some councils give grants to people on a low income towards the cost of repairs or improvements to their home.

For more information
Age Concern England Factsheet 13 *Older home owners: financial help with repairs and adaptations.*

Description
Fuel bills and telephone charges

You may be able to get a grant for insulation and draughtproofing. Some people are eligible for assistance with telephone charges.

For more information
Age Concern England Factsheet 1 *Help with heating.* Age Concern England Factsheet 28 *Help with telephones.*

Description
Help with health costs

If you receive Income Support you can get free prescriptions, dental treatment and sight tests and help towards glasses. If you do not receive Income Support you may still apply for help by filling in form HC1.

For more information
Department of Health leaflet HC11 *Are you entitled to help with health costs?* Age Concern England Factsheet 5 *Dental care in retirement.*

What happens if the person is in hospital?

The State pension and social security benefits may be affected if the person receiving them stays in hospital for more than six weeks (four weeks for some benefits, such as Attendance Allowance). How much they are reduced depends on the person's circumstances, but Housing Benefit can be paid for a year if the admission to hospital is considered to be temporary. Payment of benefits should resume in full for any time spent at home and on discharge from hospital.

For more *i*nformation

i *Your Rights*, published annually by Age Concern Books (details on p 117), a comprehensive guide to money benefits for older people.

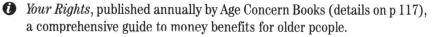

Making a Will

A Will makes it easier for relatives to carry out someone's wishes after they die. If a person dies without making a Will, he or she is said to have died intestate and their estate (all their money, property and other possessions) is divided up according to a set of predetermined rules. There may also be delays and complications in sorting out the estate. Although it may be hard to broach the subject of making a Will with your relative, if you choose the right moment, it may actually put her mind at rest.

Unless the Will is very straightforward, you should consult a solicitor. The Citizens Advice Bureau (CAB) can help you to choose a good local solicitor and may even run a free legal advice session. You will find the local CAB in the telephone directory. If you go to a solicitor directly always ask what the cost will be before the session.

Drawing up a Will yourself

If you do not use a solicitor, here are some guidelines for preparing a Will:

■ Make sure at the beginning that you say that this Will revokes all others (even if you have never made a Will before), otherwise your heirs may wonder if you have left other instructions in another Will.

■ Decide who will be your executors – the people named in the Will to deal with (administer) your affairs.

■ Choose whom you want to be the main beneficiary or beneficiaries of your estate (a beneficiary is someone who benefits from a Will). They will receive the remainder of your estate (the residue) after any other legacies have been paid.

■ Be precise – put the full name and relationship to you of any beneficiary and full details about any possessions.

■ Make provision in case any beneficiary dies before you do.

For more *i*nformation

ℹ Age Concern England Factsheet 7 *Making your Will.*

ℹ Age Concern England Factsheet 14 *Probate: dealing with someone's estate.*

ℹ *Wills and Probate, What to Do when Someone Dies* and *Will Pack,* all published by the Consumers' Association, 2 Marylebone Road, London NW1 4DF. Tel: 0171-830 6000. (These do not apply to the situation in Scotland.)

ℹ The **Alzheimer's Disease Society** (address on p 109) has a list of solicitors (LawNet) it can recommend to deal with legal and financial problems arising from dementia.

Making a 'living will'

One of the most difficult aspects of caring for someone in the advanced stages of dementia is taking decisions on their behalf. When it comes to decisions about medical treatment, it helps enormously if you have been able to discuss with your relative what her wishes would be before she became too ill.

A 'living will' or 'advance directive', as it is otherwise known, is a statement made by someone *before* they become seriously ill about the kind of medical treatment they would wish to receive or to refuse at the end of life. Although still the subject of some debate, an advance directive is now considered to be legally binding in English law, provided it is clear that the person making it understood the consequences of the request. In Scotland, the legal position is still unclear.

If the person you care for chooses to make a living will, it is a good idea to review it from time to time while she is still able to do so, and to make changes if she so wishes.

There is no fixed form for a living will, providing the person making it shows that she is fully capable of making a decision and that she understands that death may be the consequence of refusing treatment. The Voluntary Euthanasia Society (address on p 113) has produced its own advance directive. A small charge is made to non-members for a set of forms, guidance notes and an emergency medical card.

Health care proxy

'Best interests'

There is little doubt that decisions made on behalf of a person without capacity should be made in their best interests. In determining a person's best interests, regard should be given to the following factors:

■ the past and present wishes and feelings of the person concerned and the factors the person would consider if able to do so;

■ the need to permit and encourage the person to participate, or improve her ability to participate, as fully as possible in anything done for and any decision affecting her;

■ the views of other people whom it is appropriate and practical to consult about the person's wishes and feelings and what would be in her best interests; and

■ whether the purpose for which any action or decision is required can be as effectively achieved in a manner less restrictive of the person's freedom of action.

However, responsibility for diagnosing and determining the nature of medical treatment lies with an individual, qualified medical practitioner (doctor).

6 How caring affects you

Distress and emotional pain are understandable and appropriate reactions to watching someone who has dementia. Family members may feel grief, anger and despair at the same time as love and compassion. Sometimes feelings may be so strong that you feel out of control; at other times you may feel empty and unable to feel anything.

Emotions, and the way you express emotions, vary from one person to another and will largely reflect the relationship you had with your relative before he became ill. This chapter discusses some of the feelings you may experience and ways of dealing with them.

Anne

'Living with someone with dementia is mind-bending.'

'I had seven years, long, sad, lonely years. You think you are going to wake up and it's only a dream and you wonder how that happy life, that wonderful man, has changed so. I still feel it is the same awful nightmare, he didn't deserve that, he'd do anything for anyone, why did he have to suffer? I just can't bear to talk about a God any more.

'At first you try to hide it away from everyone and show a cheerful face. With someone suffering from dementia and assessments at the local mental health hospital, you feel a bit ashamed it has happened to your husband. But other patients were doctors and solicitors so it gave me some insight into what these sad-looking patients were like before this illness struck them.

'Living with someone with dementia is mind-bending – especially when they are doing strange things all day. Eric didn't want to talk and it was just me for hours on end – no one to converse with, chat about a TV pro-gramme or what's in the paper or who I met out shopping. That I found particularly hard to bear.

'I was fortunate to be on the telephone: family and friends would ring up in the evening but that was hard too. They would ask "How are you?" or usually "How is Eric?" I would say "OK" when honestly he wasn't and I was feeling dreadful and at my wits' end. I never knew (and to this day don't know) if Eric understood what I was saying – so I always made a point of being considerate and never said anything on the phone to hurt his feel-ings or something I felt it better he didn't hear.

'It is this not knowing what they can understand that is hard to come to terms with.'

How you feel as a carer

Anne's feelings while caring for her husband illustrate the over-whelming conflict of emotions which a carer can feel while coping with the practicalities of day-to-day caring. Her love for her hus-band (as he was before the illness) lived on, but it was accompanied by the sadness of knowing he was lost to her. She felt anger at the situation – and at God for letting this terrible thing happen. She felt shame and embarrassment for her husband but was also fiercely protective and considered his feelings above her own need for support. Daily losses added to her social isolation and the sense of 'not knowing' how much her husband could understand only added to her loneliness.

Anne's story may or may not ring bells for you, but it shows the difficulties of managing quite different feelings at the same time. This chapter is organised under headings, but your experience may feel very much more confused. You may, for example, have strong feelings of love and protectiveness towards your relative at the same time as feeling extremely angry with him. The way you manage your feelings is a personal matter, but it is important to sort out *what* you are feeling. If you do not recognise the source of your emotions, they may affect your own ability to make wise decisions or you may become ill yourself.

Feeling protective

Caring for someone with dementia may be physically exhausting, but it is often the mental exhaustion that carers find the most difficult to manage. This may start quite early on in the illness, since a large part of the effort of caring at this stage is often devoted to protecting the ill person from the awareness of his own declining powers.

Many carers become expert at providing care in such a way that the person is not aware of being cared for. You may be eating meals that are barely edible or jokingly dismissing memory lapses as 'just Mum's way'. Preserving the person's self-esteem and feeling of independence is often an act of love on the part of the relative or partner, but it can contribute to problems of isolation.

Nancy

'I think the first year you try to hide it, don't you? I'd answer for Frank if we were talking to somebody – you get over-protective, you stick up for your husband. When he couldn't get his words out I'd say them for him. My husband was taken into hospital for a prostate operation. When he was out of bed they couldn't find him, he'd wandered off and that brought it out into the open. Once it was out it was a great relief.'

For Nancy, it came as a relief when her husband's illness became evident to others because then she felt able to accept help with the situation. When you are trying to remain positive and to hold on to the things your relative is still able to do, it can be hard to ask for help and advice without feeling you are giving in or somehow betraying him. Many carers find they are constantly 'backstopping' to avert the next crisis.

May

'He insists on having money in his pocket – it's his independence and I don't want to take that away from him. But he doesn't know the difference between £20s, £10s and £5s. The other day he paid £40 in the greengrocers for a few veg. Luckily people know him round here but I worry about unscrupulous characters. So now I just make sure there aren't any big notes. I've put a card in his pocket with his name and address on because he's had a few falls in the street, but I didn't tell him, he wouldn't like it. I don't like doing things without my husband's knowledge, but I have to take this on myself now. You just have to find ways and means of doing things without creating waves.'

May found that with this new need to 'protect' her husband her relationship with him also changed. After 50 years of a peaceful marriage, they started to argue.

May

'He thinks I've got aggressive towards him. No doubt I have. His time clock is going wrong and last night he got into bed with his shoes on. I turned over and said, "You can stop that lark for a start." He's always been a very precise man, he worked in a drawing office. His standards were very high, but they've gone down with a bang.'

Living with loss

Anne

'To us wives, husbands and partners, it is like an ongoing bereavement. After all, you have lost the one you love. This is bad enough, but this dreadful thing is happening to them. I often felt as if I had gone and got some complete stranger with dreadful habits and behaviour off the street and was forced to look after him. I just couldn't believe I was actually in this situation and not knowing how long it was likely to continue.'

Pat

'At times he will look at me with such a lost look I am overwhelmed with a feeling of sadness and loss and just have to hold him tight.'

Perhaps the hardest part of caring for a person with dementia is the loss and sadness you inevitably feel. Loss of a relationship that you once had, loss of a companion or friend, sadness at seeing a capable, lively person lose his zest for life and his ability to do quite simple things. Each new loss can leave you feeling sad and discouraged, and these feelings can be very hard to bear. The grief you feel may be every bit as strong as the feelings another person has when someone dies. These feelings may come and go, alternating with times of optimism. Then another deterioration occurs and you are thrown into despair again.

There is no easy way to deal with these difficult feelings, but knowing that they are normal and that others have gone through the same reactions may be some comfort. This does not mean that you have to carry on coping with an unbearable situation where you feel trapped and unable to manage any longer.

Shame and embarrassment

Jim

'Her table manners are dreadful now. She would have been shocked to know she has come to this.'

Anne

'We had one day when Eric repeatedly kept taking his trousers down in the sitting room. I found that embarrassing.'

As your relative's confusion becomes more evident to outsiders and some of his behaviour becomes antisocial, you may suffer severe embarrassment. It can help if you explain to others what is happening. Try not to let embarrassment get in the way of seeing people: good friends should be able to tolerate changes in behaviour and understand that you need to continue to keep in contact with them.

Loneliness and isolation

Doris

'My mother was, until the day of the "crisis", very active and enjoyed cooking an evening meal. Afterwards she could not remember the layout of the flat and still asks where rooms are. She cannot remember my father who died 20 years ago and has no recall of my birth or childhood. The days and weeks after her diagnosis cannot be described adequately. I was alone with a stranger. Not knowing how to cope is frightening. Perhaps the worst of all is not being able to touch and love someone who is so dear. Any attempt to show affection is met with, "Don't be so silly, go away."'

There may be times when you feel terribly alone, particularly if you were very close to your relative before the illness. The changes in his personality may be very hurtful to you and the demands of adapting to such a different person may make you feel tense and anxious. In addition, you may have to take on practical tasks that were previously your relative's responsibility: cooking, DIY or paying bills.

Hard as it is to make the effort when you feel miserable, don't cut yourself off from family or friends. Ask for help when you need it and let them know how you feel – they may not realise how difficult you are finding things unless you tell them. You might find that talking to other people in the same situation helps you to feel less alone (see pp 35–37).

Anger and irritation

John

'She would aggravate me so much sometimes that I would get really cross and I had to go out into the hall to cool down. Then she'd come out and put her arms round me and say, "I'm sorry, I didn't mean to be like that." It would be her old self showing through.'

Nancy

'Frank doesn't get moods. He's very quiet, but he can never find anything. He will put something down and spend two hours looking for it. I say to him "Put your blue coat on" and he will reply "I haven't got a blue coat." You can stand it for a few hours, then you just want to scream.'

However well you are adapting to the demands of a person with dementia, you are almost certain to feel anger and irritation at times, especially when you are tired and under stress. It can help to remember that the behaviour that makes you feel angry is caused by the illness, and is not directed at you personally. But don't feel guilty if you do lose your temper and exchange cross words. Look back to pages 64–67 and see if there are any ways you can avoid a confrontation in the future.

It may not be the confused person who makes you feel angry: you may legitimately feel anger at the insensitivity of professionals or the lack of practical services to help you. Beth looks after her 92-year-old mother, who is blind, incontinent and barely mobile:

Beth

'Carers live on a knife edge of uncertainty and no one official ever says "You're doing a good job!" Just an invisible resource to be used up like a tube of toothpaste – that's us.'

Carers like Beth have been the backbone of the campaign to improve the rights of carers. Anger can be a potent force for change if you have an outlet for it. If you feel you want to contribute to campaigning for a better deal for carers, contact the Carers National Association (address on p 110).

Occasionally carers reach the point where they are physically aggressive towards the person with dementia. This is a sign that you need help. Speak to a trusted friend or professional or contact one of the organisations listed later in the chapter (p 107).

Eve

'I cared for my mother for several years. She was a sweet lady but ah! so trying. She had taken Nembutal sleeping tablets since she was in her 40s, then when she was about 90 they withdrew them. My doctor told me it was the worst thing that could have happened to her as she was addicted. She became so very difficult, awake all night and sleeping most of the day. One night I got quite desperate. She could not get upstairs, so I slept on a camp-bed in the lounge and she was on the settee. I picked up a cushion to put over her face – she was so restless and I couldn't get any rest either. Some power, God I think, stopped me, fortunately. She said to me, "Go on, do it, you'll be charged with murder!"'

Uncertainty

Jill

'Nearly every day is a crisis with my mother-in-law – from the ones you can laugh at to the more serious ones like boiling a kettle on the gas stove then forgetting why she did it, leaving the kitchen full of steam.'

Living with someone who has dementia can be nerve-racking. You never know what is going to happen next and you need to be alert to the possible dangers. You are also living with the uncertainty of the illness itself. Everybody with dementia responds in a different way, and you can never be sure what the next 'stage' will bring, or how long the caring will go on. Professionals can only tell you what might happen, but in the meantime the physical strain of caring continues.

Joyce

'For me, it is the tedium and the length of time this "caring" has been going on. My husband is 68 and has had Parkinson's disease for 12 years. Originally he was diagnosed as a depressive but following a brain scan he was diagnosed as having Alzheimer's disease. He has hallucinations and his mind returns to different periods in his life, for instance his office life, when presumably I am his secretary. He is "childlike" if he wants something: he wants it immediately and shouts. He is quite wily, so that if I am upstairs he will find excuses to keep me going up and down. Either he is going to faint, or he wants to go to the toilet, or he can't get himself out of a chair – all quite valid reasons for calling me – so that I can't take chances by ignoring them.'

The difficulty of looking after someone when you do not know what they understand can make you feel helpless or resentful. Your best efforts to look after your relative may be met with little thanks or positive hostility.

Lucy

'The shock of my own mother not knowing me was horrifying. I was called "you", and even now I am treated as someone who is there to cook, clean, shop and more often than not make a nuisance of myself and demand she gets up, dress, eat and behave in a way she always has done, when she would rather be left alone.'

Try not to bottle up your feelings. Other families caring for a person with dementia will understand what you are going through. Although nobody can tell you what the future holds, it can help to find out about the illness and its possible course. You have made a start by reading this book, and you can find out more by contacting the relevant charity or voluntary organisation (addresses on pp 109–113).

Exhaustion

Ben

'Often I could just lie down from tiredness, from the pain of worry and the frustration of it all. But I gather my strength again and carry on.'

Don't wait until you are desperate or ill to ask for help. Looking after a person with dementia is exhausting and you need to take breaks and have a life of your own if you are going to be able to help the person you care for. Look back to pages 54–57 for more about how to get a break from caring.

You may be having broken nights if you live with a person who has dementia. Take the line of least resistance, doing what you can to get as much rest as possible while ensuring your relative is safe.

Alice

'We live in a bungalow that has been extended to accommodate my 86-year-old mother on the ground floor while my husband and I have a bedroom and bathroom upstairs. We now make sure all the doors on the ground floor are locked at night, including the bathroom (fortunately we also have a separate WC which of course remains open). Our central heating is on low all night. At first, I would go dashing downstairs if I heard a sound and I seemed to sleep in a state of semi-alertness. Now, I have decided that I will only go down if she actually calls out. I now find that I am sleeping better and have decided that it doesn't really matter if now and again my mother is dressed, semi-dressed or even up when we go to wake her.'

Love, compassion and humour

Lesley

'She has to be spoon fed each meal, she cannot walk, she cannot converse – although I am convinced she knows what is being said. She is so pleasant and not in any pain, and is quite content with me.'

Jim

'We have been together 58 years, years of love and happiness. I have been her carer for three years and am happy to be able to do it.'

Some people are able to find new ways of expressing and sharing their love in the midst of the pain of seeing a loved one becoming ill. This is a great gift, but your love for the person should not prevent you admitting your need for help. As the person becomes more dependent, you need to ask for and to accept help for the good of both of you.

Humour is often a wonderful way of defusing the anxiety and tension that can build up when you are caring for someone with dementia. The illness does have its funny side and there is nothing wrong with enjoying a laugh at some of the more bizarre events that punctuate your days of caring.

Dave

'Before I went to work in the morning I would give her breakfast. To give her a little job to do, I would get her into the kitchen and sit her at the table and ask her to make me a sandwich to take with me and to put the cat's breakfast in her dish. I remember once, when tea break came at work, trying to eat my Whiskas-filled sandwich. I often wonder if Fluffy enjoyed her cheese and pickle.'

Other members of the family

When a person develops dementia, everyone in the family is affected in some way. Young children and teenagers are often very patient, understanding and loving with a relative who has dementia. They may cope better than adults. Even if this is the case, it is important to realise that the situation has a profound effect on their lives. If you have young children they need plenty of reassurance and physical affection to show that you still love them, however worried and preoccupied you may seem. Try to make regular time to talk to children about what is happening and allow them to talk about their own feelings of fear, grief, bewilderment or anger.

Teenage children may resent the demands your relative makes on you or they may be embarrassed by his behaviour. Some will want to help and take the load away from you by hiding their own problems. However they show it, most will also experience feelings of loss and pain as the illness progresses. Such mixed feelings are hard to manage for an adult, and for an adolescent who has other changes and uncertainties to contend with, these can be difficult times. Make sure your teenager understands what is happening and is involved in important decisions. Make sure, too, that you express your appreciation for any help your child offers and for the effort they make to talk things through with you. If you are concerned about a teenage child and think he or she needs further support, your local Alzheimer's Disease Society, carers' group or community psychiatric nurse may be able to provide an independent listening ear.

Your partner will also be affected when you are looking after a parent or parent-in-law with dementia. If the person is living in the same house, your relationship with your partner will be severely tested. It is natural to take out your frustrations and anger on those you are closest to. In addition, the sheer effort of caring can have repercussions on a relationship. You may be more stretched financially, you will certainly be more tired, and it may be hard to find time to talk, go out or make love. There are no easy answers, but it is important to enter the situation with open eyes and to plan time when you can be with your partner without your ill parent in order to enjoy your relationship together.

For more *i*nformation

ⓘ Alzheimer's Disease Society Advice Sheet 8 *Grief and bereavement.*

ⓘ Alzheimer's Disease Society Advice Sheet 16 *Telling the children.*

ⓘ Alzheimer's Disease Society Advice Sheet 17 *Dealing with guilt.*

Coping with caring

As a carer, you need plenty of help and support. You *have* to put yourself and your own needs first if you are to continue caring.

Meg

'I used to sit and cry, not knowing which way to turn, and even contemplated suicide. His brother and sister-in-law were in London, both ill, and his sister and husband were in Wales and didn't believe what I told them!'

If things have reached the point where

- you need alcohol or pills to get you through the day *or*
- you are contemplating suicide *or*
- you are losing weight and feeling unwell

you *must* find someone who you can talk to who will give you a different perspective on the situation. If you do not have a friend, relative or sympathetic doctor you can turn to, try contacting one of these organisations (all addresses and phone numbers on pp 109–113):

- the Samaritans;
- the Alzheimer's Disease Society (or the organisation that is most closely linked to the illness which is causing the dementia);
- the Carers National Association.

These DOs and DON'Ts may help:

Do look after your own health. Don't dismiss potentially serious symptoms like high blood pressure, constant headaches and feeling dizzy. See your own GP about health problems, and don't be afraid to mention psychological or emotional problems.

Don't wait until you are desperate to ask for help. Finding out about services that can support you does not mean that you are being disloyal to the person you care for.

Do find someone to talk to to share your feelings, worries and fears (see pp 35–37).

Do explain to friends and neighbours what is happening, both to save you embarrassment and so that they can offer appropriate help.

Don't cut yourself off from friends and relatives. Keep them informed of changes and tell them what they can do to help.

Don't blame yourself if you occasionally lose your temper or feel overwhelmed by the situation.

Do find out about respite care, so that you can have a break from time to time (see pp 54–57).

Do make contact with other carers. They could be your lifeline (see pp 35–36 on carers' groups).

Don't be afraid to ask for the help you need, from social services, your doctor or your family.

Don't think you have to go on caring for ever. As your relative's dementia progresses, you may feel that residential or nursing home care is the only solution.

Don't feel guilty about it if you do make this decision.

Useful addresses

Accountant of Court
Information about curator bonis in Scotland.

2 Parliament House
Parliament Square
Edinburgh EH1 1RQ
Tel: 0131-225 2595

AIDS helpline

0800 567 123
(confidential – 24 hours)

Alzheimer Scotland – Action on Dementia
Information and support for people with dementia and their carers in Scotland. Supports a network of carers support groups.

22 Drumsheugh Gardens
Edinburgh EH3 7RN
Tel: 0131-243 1453
24-hour helpline:
0800 317 817

Alzheimer's Disease Society
Information, support and advice about caring for someone with Alzheimer's disease. They can also direct you to regional and local groups.

Gordon House
10 Greencoat Place
London SW1P 1PH
Tel: 0171-306 0606

AVERT
AIDS Education and Research Trust, which produces a range of medical self-help booklets.

11–13 Denne Parade
Horsham
West Sussex RH12 1JD
Tel: 01403 210202

British Association for Counselling
For a list of counsellors and organisations in your area.

1 Regent Place
Rugby
Warwickshire CV21 2PJ
Tel: 01788 578328

British Federation of Care Home Proprietors
Members must meet the standards of care set by the Federation. Can provide lists of homes; it also produces a useful checklist of questions to ask called How to choose a good care home.

Elmsdale House
Wood Street North
Alfreton
Derbyshire DE55 7GR
Tel: 01773 831966

British Red Cross Society
Can loan home aids for disabled people. Local branches in many areas.

9 Grosvenor Crescent
London SW1X 7EJ
Tel: 0171-235 5454

CANDID (Counselling and Diagnosis in Dementia)
Offers a counselling service aimed at younger people with dementia.

National Hospital for
Neurology and
Neurosurgery
Queens Square
London WC1N 3BG
Tel: 0171-837 3611
ext. 3855

Carers National Association
Provides information and advice if you are looking after someone, whether in your own home or at a distance. Can put you in touch with other carers and carers' groups in your area.

20–25 Glasshouse Yard
London EC1A 4JS
Tel: 0171-490 8818
CarersLine: 0171-490 8898

Chest, Heart and Stroke (Scotland)
Aims to improve the quality of life for people in Scotland affected by chest, heart or stoke illness through medical research, health promotion, advice, information, and the provision of services.

65 North Castle Street
Edinburgh EH2 3LT
Tel: 0131-225 6963

Continence Foundation
Advice and information about whom to contact with incontinence problems.

Doughty Street
London WC1N 2PH
Tel: 0171-404 6875

Counsel and Care
*Aims to visit every registered private
and voluntary residential and nursing
home in the London area. Can also
offer advice on funding for residential
care, and a range of factsheets.*

Twyman House
16 Bonny Street
London NW1 9PG
Tel: 0171-485 1566
(10.30 am–4.00 pm)

Court of Protection
*If you need to take over the affairs of
someone who is mentally incapable
in England or Wales.*

Public Trust Office
Stewart House
24 Kingsway
London WC2B 6JX
Tel: 0171-664 7300

Crossroads Care
*For a care attendant to come into
your home and look after the person
you care for.*

10 Regent Place
Rugby
Warwickshire CV21 2PN
Tel: 01788 573653

Disability Scotland
*For people in Scotland who need
advice or information about disability.*

Princes House
5 Shandwick Place
Edinburgh EH2 4RG
Tel: 0131-229 8632

Elderly Accommodation Counsel
*Has a national register of
accommodation in the voluntary and
private sectors suitable for older
people. Can provide a computer
printout of information directly to
older people or their relations.*

46A Chiswick High Road
London W4 1SZ
Tel: 0181-995 8320/
742 1182

Help the Aged
*Provides free advice and information
for older people, their relatives,
friends and carers. Seniorline is a
free information and advice
service.*

16–18 St James's Walk
London EC1R 0BE
Tel: 0171-253 0253
Seniorline: 0800 650 065
Minicom: 0800 269 626

Huntington's Disease Association
*Information and advice for carers
of people with Huntington's disease
(Huntington's chorea).*

108 Battersea High Street
London SW11 3HP
Tel: 0171-223 7000

Incontinence Information Helpline
*Information and advice about
managing incontinence, and how to
contact your nearest continence adviser.*

Tel: 0191-213 0050
9 am–6 pm Monday–Friday

Local Government Ombudsman
*If you want to make a complaint
about the local authority.*

21 Queen Anne's Gate
London SW1H 9BU
Tel: 0171-915 3210

**MIND (National Association for
Mental Health)**
*Publishes books, reports and leaflets.
It aims to help people understand
what is meant by 'mental illness',
to make people aware of their rights,
and to create a debate about how
mental health services are run.*

Granta House
15–19 Broadway
London E15 4BQ
Tel: 0181-519 2122

National Care Homes Association
*An umbrella body for local
associations of private care homes.
Can put you in touch with homes
in your area which meet the
standards set by the Association.*

Martin House
3rd Floor
84–86 Gray's Inn Road
London WC1X 8BQ
Tel: 0171-831 7090

**Office of Care and Protection
(Northern Ireland)**
*If you need to take over the affairs
of someone who is mentally
incapable in Northern Ireland.*

Royal Courts of Justice
PO Box 410
Chichester Street
Belfast BT1 3JF

Parkinson's Disease Society
*Support and information for
relatives and carers of someone
with Parkinson's disease.*

22 Upper Woburn Place
London WC1H ORA
Tel: 0171-383 3513

Public Trust Office

See Court of Protection

**Registered Nursing Home
Association**
*Can give you information about
registered nursing homes in your
area which meet the standards
set by the Association.*

Calthorpe House
Hagley Road
Edgbaston
Birmingham B16 8QY
Tel: 0121-454 2511

Relatives Association
Advice, information and support for
relatives of people in a residential
or nursing home. Produces leaflets
and offers a listening ear and
opportunities to join or form local
groups.

5 Tavistock Place
London WC1H 9SS
Tel: 0171-916 6055

Samaritans
Someone to talk to if you are in
despair.

See your local telephone
directory.

**Scottish Association for Mental
Health (SAMH)**
SAMH is the largest voluntary
organisation in mental health in
Scotland providing projects, support
and research.

Cumbrae House
15 Carlton Place
Glagow G5 9JP
Tel: 0141-568 7000

Stroke Association
Information and advice if you are
caring for someone who has had a
stroke.

CHSA House
Whitecross Street
London EC1Y 8JJ
Tel: 0171-490 7999

Voluntary Euthanasia Society
Provides forms for an advance
directive plus guidance notes.

13 Prince of Wales Terrace
London W8 5PG
Tel: 0171-937 7770

About Age Concern

Caring for someone who has dementia is one of a wide range of publications produced by Age Concern England, the National Council on Ageing. Age Concern cares about all older people and believes later life should be fulfilling and enjoyable. For too many this is impossible. As the leading charitable movement in the UK concerned with ageing and older people, Age Concern finds effective ways to change that situation.

Where possible, we enable older people to solve problems themselves, providing as much or as little support as they need. Our network of 1,400 local groups, supported by 250,000 volunteers, provides community-based services such as lunch clubs, day centres and home visiting.

Nationally, we take a lead role in campaigning, parliamentary work, policy analysis, research, specialist information and advice provision, and publishing. Innovative programmes promote healthier lifestyles and provide older people with opportunities to give the experience of a lifetime back to their communities.

Age Concern is dependent on donations, covenants and legacies.

Age Concern England
1268 London Road
London SW16 4ER
Tel: 0181-765 7200

Age Concern Cymru
4th Floor
1 Cathedral Road
Cardiff CF1 9SD
Tel: 01222 371566

Age Concern Scotland
113 Rose Street
Edinburgh EH2 3DT
Tel: 0131-220 3345

Age Concern Northern Ireland
3 Lower Crescent
Belfast BT7 1NR
Tel: 01232 245729

Other books in this series

The Carer's Handbook: What to do and who to turn to
Marina Lewycka
At some point in their lives millions of people find themselves suddenly responsible for organising the care of an older person with a health crisis. All too often such carers have no idea what services are available or who can be approached for support. This book is designed to act as a first point of reference in just such an emergency, signposting readers on to many more detailed, local sources of advice.
£6.99 0-86242-262-0

Caring for someone who is dying
Penny Mares
Confronting the knowledge that a loved one is going to die soon is always a moment of crisis. And the pain of the news can be compounded by the need to take responsibility for the care and support given in the last months and weeks. This book attempts to help readers cope with their emotions, identify the needs which the situation creates and make the practical arrangements necessary to ensure that the passage through the period is as smooth as possible.
£6.99 0-86242-260-4

Finding and paying for residential and nursing home care
Marina Lewycka
Acknowledging that an older person needs residential care often represents a major crisis for family and friends. Feelings of guilt and betrayal invariably compound the difficulties faced in identifying a suitable care home and sorting out the financial arrangements. This book provides a practical step-by-step guide to the decisions which have to be made and the help which is available.
£6.99 0-86242-261-2

Caring for someone who has had a stroke
Philip Coyne with Penny Mares

Although 100,000 people in Britain will have a stroke this year, many people are still confused about what stroke actually means. This book is designed to help carers understand stroke and its immediate aftermath. It contains extensive information on hospital discharge, providing care, rehabilitation, and adjustment to life at home.

£6.99 0-86242-264-7

Choices for the carer of an elderly relative
Marina Lewycka

Being a carer may mean many different things – from living at a distance and keeping a check on things by telephone to taking on a full-time caring role. This book looks at the choices facing someone whose parent or other relative needs care. It helps readers look at their own circumstances and their own priorities and decide what is the best role for themselves – as well as the person being cared for.

£6.99 0-86242-263-9

Caring for Someone with an Alcohol Problem
Mike Ward

When drinking becomes a problem, the consequences for the carer can be physically and emotionally exhausting. This book will help anyone who lives with or cares for a problem drinker, with particular emphasis on caring for an older problem drinker.

£6.99 0-86242-227-2

Caring for Someone at a Distance
Julie Spencer-Cingöz

With people now living longer, sooner or later, we are likely to find ourselves looking after a loved one or a friend – often at a distance. This book will help you to identify the needs and priorities that have to be addressed.

£6.99 0-86242-228-0

Publications from Age Concern Books

Health and care

The Community Care Handbook: The reformed system explained (2nd edition)
Barbara Meredith

The provision of care in the community is changing as a result of recent legislation. Written by one of the country's foremost experts, this book explains in practical terms the background to the reforms, what they are, how they are working and who they affect.

£13.99 0-86242-171-3

Dementia Care: A handbook for residential and day care
Alan Chapman, Alan Jacques and Mary Marshall

The number of dementia sufferers requiring care is increasing continuously. Written to complement *Taking Good Care*, this practical guide for professional carers offers an understanding of the condition and provides advice on such issues as daily care, health maintenance, home design and staffing strategies.

£11.99 0-86242-128-4

Money matters

Your Rights: A guide to money benefits for older people
Sally West

A highly acclaimed annual guide to the State benefits available to older people. Contains current information on Income Support, Housing Benefit and Retirement Pensions, among other matters, and provides advice on how to claim.

For further information please telephone 0181-679 8000.

Managing Other People's Money (2nd edition)
Penny Letts
Foreword by The Master of the Court of Protection
The management of money and property is usually a personal and private matter. However, there may come a time when someone else has to take over on either a temporary or a permanent basis. This book looks at the circumstances in which such a need could arise and provides a step-by-step guide to the arrangements which have to be made.

£9.99 0-86242-250-7

If you would like to order any of these titles, please write to the address below, enclosing a cheque or money order for the appropriate amount made payable to Age Concern England. Credit card orders may be made on 0181-765 7200.

Mail Order Unit
Age Concern England
1268 London Road
London SW16 4ER

Information Line

Age Concern produces over 40 comprehensive factsheets designed to answer many of the questions older people – or those advising them – may have, on topics such as:

- finding and paying for residential and nursing home care
- money benefits
- finding help at home
- legal affairs
- making a Will
- help with heating
- raising income from your home
- transfer of assets

Age Concern offers a factsheet subscription service that presents all the factsheets in a folder, together with regular updates throughout the year. The first year's subscription currently costs £50; an annual renewal thereafter is £25.

To order your FREE factsheet list, phone 0800 00 99 66 (a free call) or write to:

Age Concern
FREEPOST (SWB 30375)
Ashburton
Devon TQ13 7ZZ

Index